STRENGTH A
IN KIDNEY FAILURE

STRENGTH AND COMPASSION IN KIDNEY FAILURE

Writings of Mildred (Barry) Friedman
Professional Kidney Patient

Forewords by

WILLEM J. KOLFF, M.D.
Distinguished Professor of Medicine and Surgery Emeritus,
University of Utah

BELDING H. SCRIBNER, M.D.
Professor of Medicine Emeritus,
University of Washington

THOMAS STARZL, M.D.
Director, Pittsburgh Transplantation Institute

Preface and Annotations by

ELI A. FRIEDMAN, M.D.

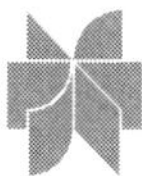

KLUWER ACADEMIC PUBLISHERS
DORDRECHT / BOSTON / LONDON

A C.I.P. Catalogue record for this book is available from the Library of Congress.

ISBN 0-7923-5235-1 (HB)
ISBN 0-7923-5236-X (PB)

Published by Kluwer Academic Publishers,
P.O. Box 17, 3300 AA Dordrecht, The Netherlands.

Sold and distributed in North, Central and South America
by Kluwer Academic Publishers,
101 Philip Drive, Norwell, MA 02061, U.S.A.

In all other countries, sold and distributed
by Kluwer Academic Publishers,
P.O. Box 322, 3300 AH Dordrecht, The Netherlands.

Printed on acid-free paper

Printed in the Netherlands

Dedication

Barry talked often of her sister Joan's magnificent gift of life. For seventeen years, Barry's every breath, activity, and plan was contingent on the restoration of renal function permitted by her sister's altruism and generosity. Of the many good and wondrous interventions that permitted Barry to see her daughters wed and hold her grandchildren, none matches the scope of Joan's organ donation. With appreciation for the extended time with Barry and for a lifetime of her love and devotion, the Friedman family dedicates this book to Joan Barrett-Lennard Hubbard.

Legends for Mildred "Barry" Friedman Photographs

Page VI

Top. Eight grandchildren starting at the top and proceeding clockwise: Karen, Davey, Lee, Ruthie, Matan, Jeremy, Sharon, and Ben. Matan was born three weeks after Barry's death but was a part of her thoughts throughout.
Bottom. Barry with large print typewriter, starting her writing career in 1976.

Page VII

Barry at various stages. Top left before contracting diabetes. Top right, her favorite schoolgirl photo.
Midleft with husband at National Kidney Foundation of New York Award Ceremony. Mid right shows two views with sister Joan, her kidney donor, as elementary school students and fifteen years following Joan's donation of a kidney.
Lower left Barry and Joan with Father Hugh Barrett-Lennard, the family titleholder and priest at London's Brompton Oratory. Father Hugh, seen here in England, flew to attend Barry's tenth and fifteenth transplant anniversary celebrations. Lower right with family during Egyptian holiday: left to right Sara, Barry, Becky, Amy, and Eli.

Page VIII

Vibrancy of Barry's social interactions. Top left with Congressman Charles Rangle. Top right with jazz giant Lionel Hampton and husband.
Early and late views of married life. Two photos from school days. Lower right, family picture during harsh days of weight loss due to Addison's disease. Daughters left to right; Becky, Sara, Amy.

Page IX

Medical powerhouse. Top, some of Barry's medical support team at her fifteenth transplant anniversary. Left to right, Joon H. Hong, Jody Blanco, Mariana M. Markell, Khalid M. H. Butt, Julius R. Berger, Francis A. L'Esperance, Jr.. Insert superimposed on top right: Barry with diabetes nurse-educator, and long-term friend Linda Cohen.
Middle row Thomas E. Starzl at Capri, Willem J. Kolff in Kampen, Holland.
Lower right George E. Schreiner in New York, Belding H. Scribner in Bavaria.

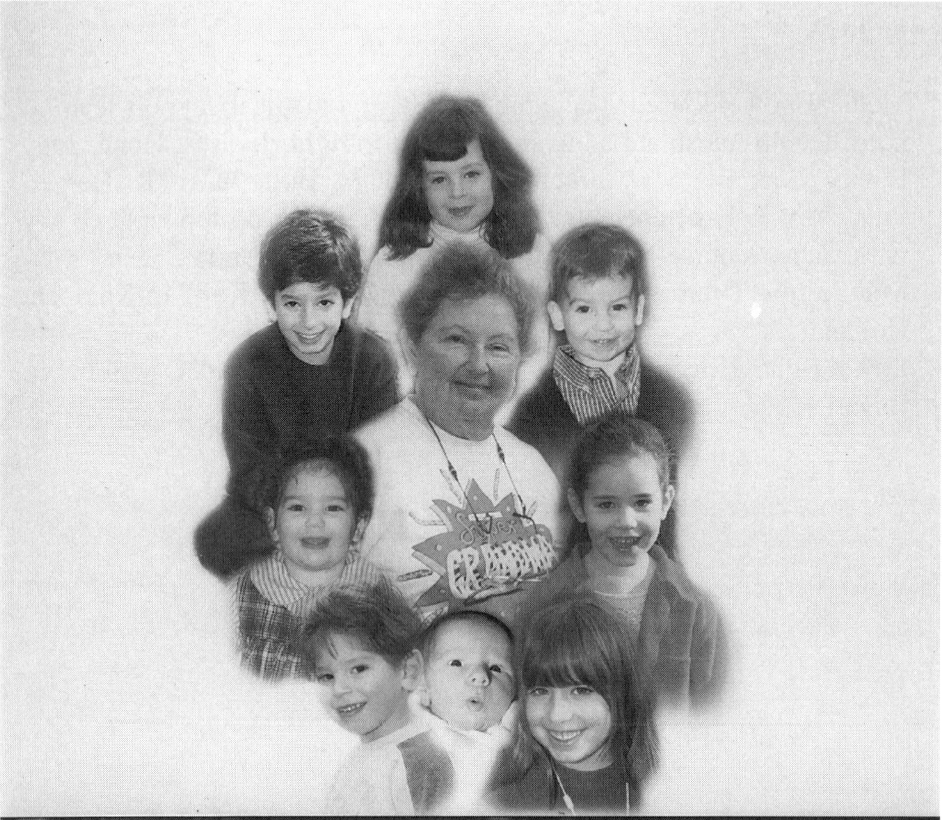

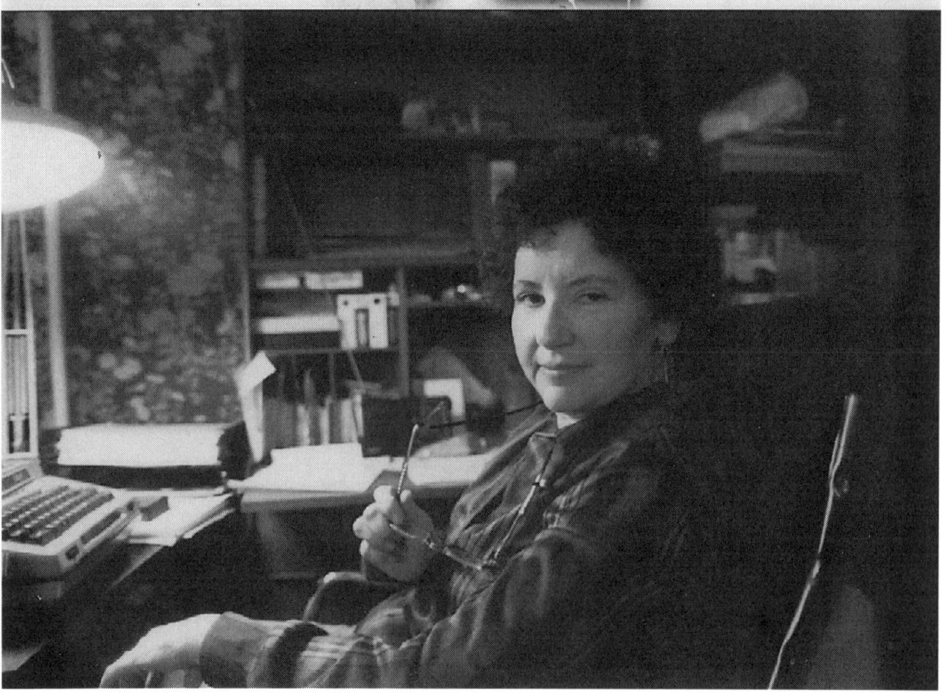

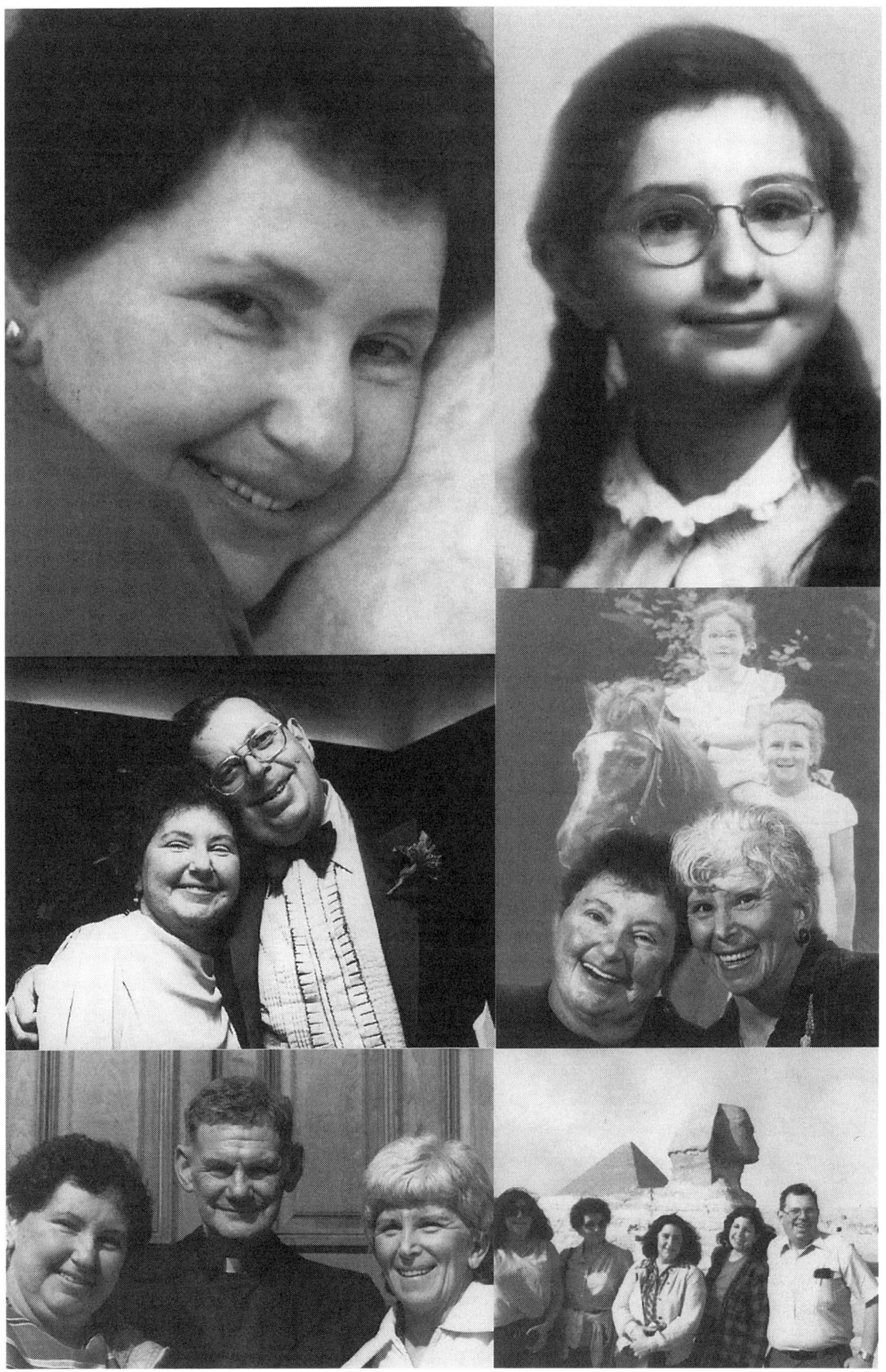

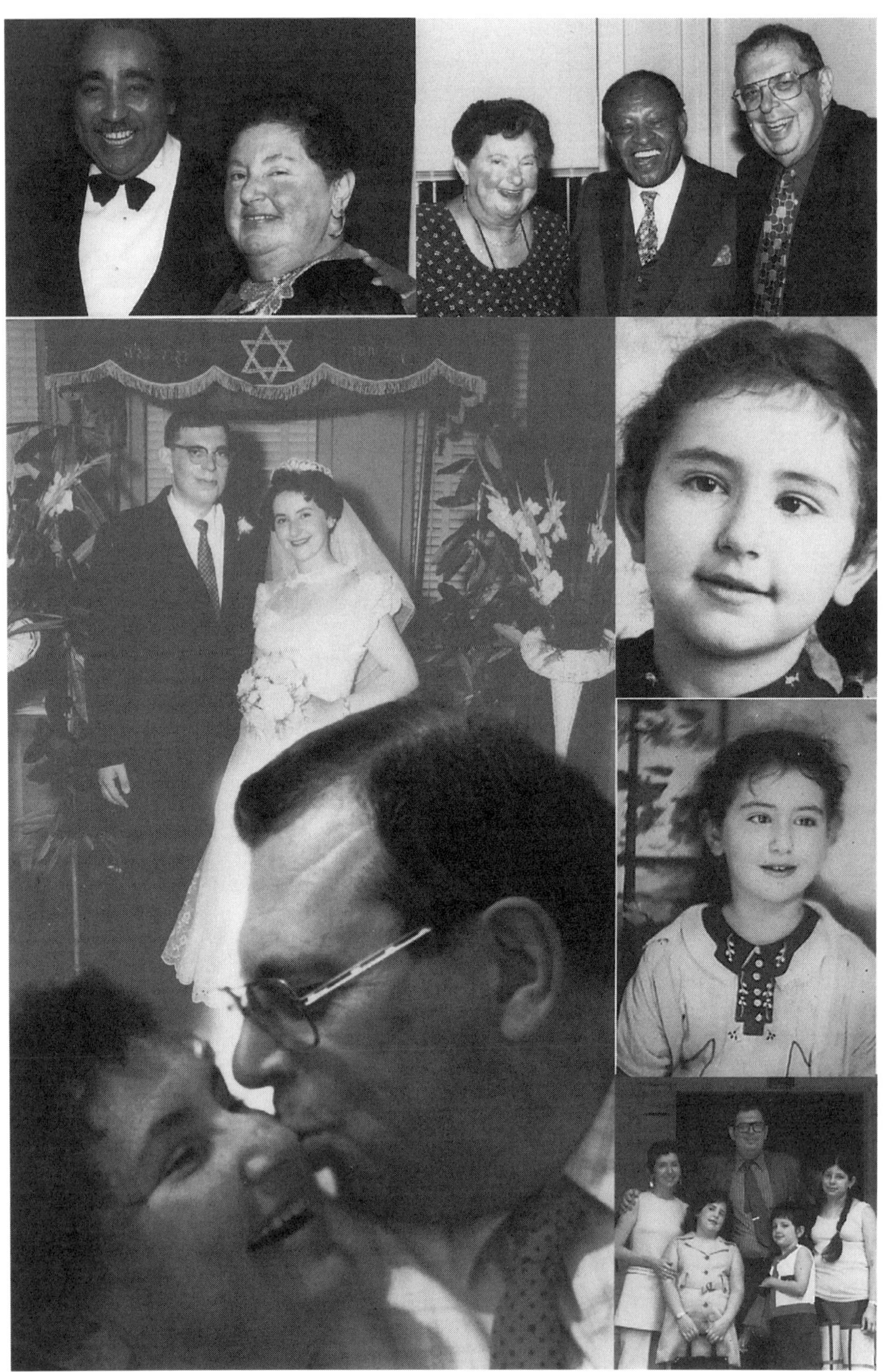

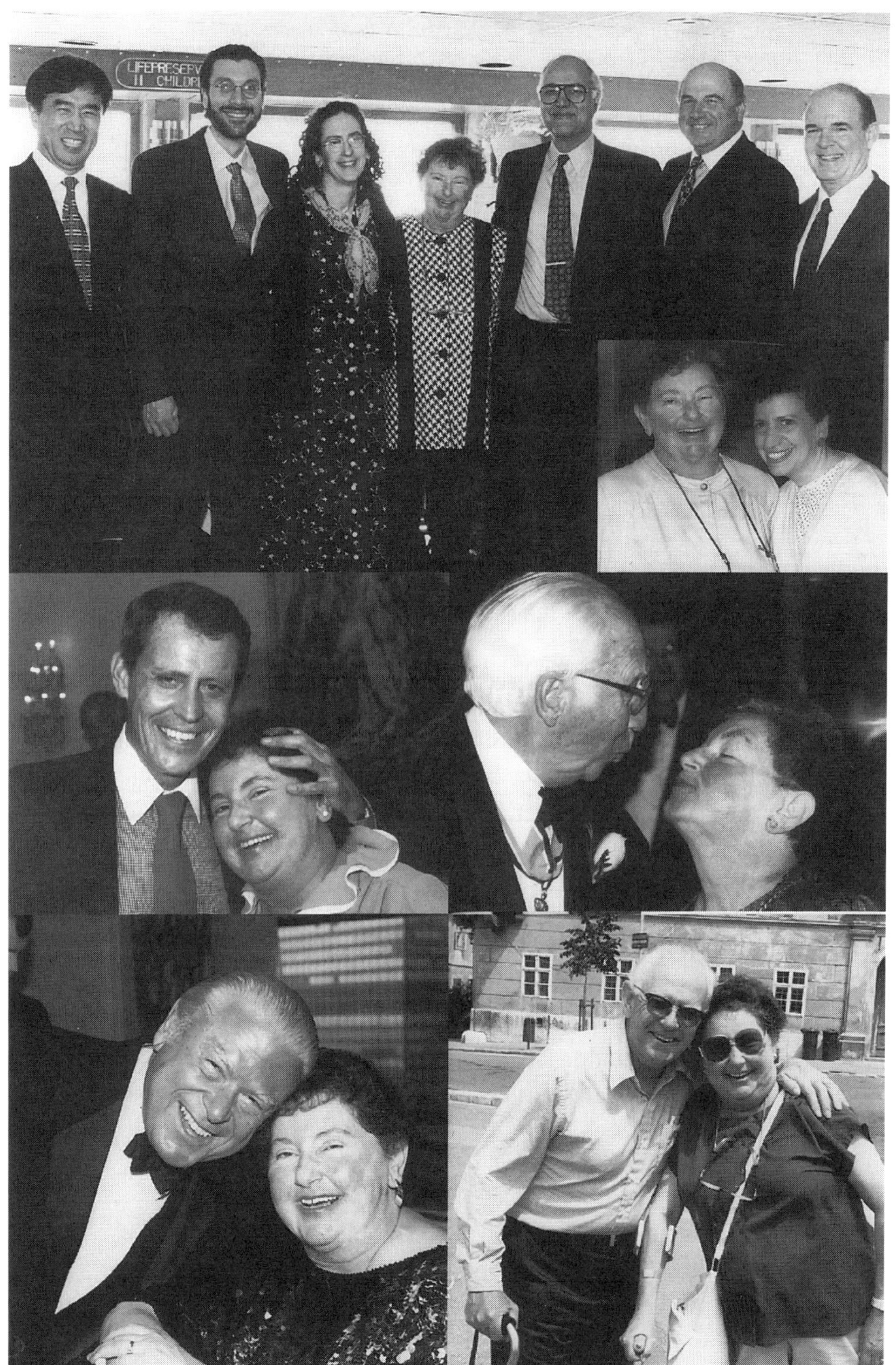

Willem J. Kolff who designed the first practical artificial kidney had frequent interaction with Barry at conferences and through their mutual support of patient organizations. When requested to prepare a forward to this book he immediately agreed and included a note with the manuscript, stating: "I have never written anything with more pleasure."

Barry

Why did I feel so wonderfully relaxed when I was sitting next to Barry Friedman in a large circle of mostly unknown people? I forgot what meeting. I forgot at what hotel. I forgot about what we talked but I will never forget the feeling of being completely content of sitting next to her. It was not because of the many common interests that we had but because of the responses we shared which was evident after half a sentence.

I am in debt to patients like Barry. Only those that benefit from the artificial kidney make our efforts worth while. It is not always that way!

I was called by a physician in Cleveland about a patient about to die from an overdose of nembutol. He assured me that she did not have a chronic depression but had taken an overdose on impulse. So, we dialyzed her. I have never heard such vile language as I had to face the next day. She had been depressed for 9 years and had spent most of the family's resources on useless psychiatrists. I had ruined her last and only chance to get to the medicine cabinet, that from now on would be locked. What right did I have to prolong her misery? I "should burn in Hell" but deserved far worse.

On the other hand, I was called by a man in a large city in the east. His wife was dying in renal failure, she had diabetes and amputation of both legs above the knees. He said that nobody wanted to dialyze her.

"Was she happy? Is her life worthwhile?"
"She is the happiest person you will ever meet and she is the joy of my life."

"How was he going to pay the hospital and the transportation?" He said that he had sued the previous physician and that he now had enough money.

I called the present physician, accepted her and she was flown to Salt Lake City.

A small person without legs is light and he carried her in his arms. She was near death; we dialyzed her immediately and she did well. Indeed, she may have been the happiest person I ever met.

What is this elixir of joy? How could Barry with a frightening medical history spread joy around her family and richly reward her husband for his skill, care, and unfaltering devotion?

She had a desire to help and her inborn gift to write communicated her happy outlook to numerous people on dialysis and others in need.

We can make artificial kidneys, and improve them, but we cannot produce la Joie de Vivre, the Lebensfreude, the Joy of Life. Barry Friedman did that. And we are all very grateful.

Pim Kolff
February 18, 1998

Belding H. Scribner forced me into a career change though he was unaware of the impact on my life of his introduction of maintenance hemodialysis. Working as a New York City Career Scientist exploring the mechanism of skin graft rejection in rabbits, I was amazed, intrigued, and genuinely attracted by Scribner's 1960 epochal demonstration that irreversible kidney failure need not mean death. Once I interviewed patients treated with repetitive hemodialysis, I was hooked. Scrib became, de facto, my mentor. Since then, dialysis has become an everyday treatment sustaining nearly one million people worldwide. For me, dialysis served as a holding therapy that kept Barry alive while her transplant was planned. I thank Scrib for his gift of life to medicine and my family.

Barry

My dear friend, Eli Friedman, gave me his usual clear assignment when he asked me to pay homage to Barry by writing this Foreword. My assignment: "What I would like from you is your view on patient activism as a survival tool."

In my view there never has been a time since 1960 when dialysis patients in the United States need to become activists on their own behalf. Let me explain my position.

I have always likened the history of insulin in the treatment of diabetics, to the history of dialysis in the treatment of chronic kidney failure. Unfortunately, I have never written about this comparison before, which is unfortunate because I should have done so and gotten invaluable input from Barry herself.

There are many similarities between diabetics and dialysis patients including the fact that the more the patients know about the treatment how and how it effects them, the better the outcome. Unfortunately, there is one vital area where this historical comparison is dissimilar: The history of insulin reveals steady improvement in outcome over the decades of the 20th century. In contrast, the patient outcomes on dialysis especially as measured by survival have tended to decline over the decades since the 1960's.

As we come to the end of this century, the outlook continues to be bleak. Unlike the diabetic in the 30's, 40's and 50's when the learning curve was the steepest, there are no institutions like the Joslin Clinic to which dialysis patients can go to really learn how to become the best possible patients. The peddling of dialysis by corporate America has become a national scandal in part because a short dialysis is a profitable dialysis, which also appeals to the uneducated patient. Most Nephrology training programs turn out Nephrologists that do not understand that chronic uremia like diabetes is a life long illness and requires unique skills to manage it.

In my view one way to try to reverse this downtrend is to form a strong, richly endowed, patient education and advocacy group with a medical and staff advisory board whose members clearly understand what good dialysis treatment is all about and how it effects survival and especially patient well-being.

Such an effort would truly honor the memory of that gallant lady, Mildred Friedman.

Belding H. Scribner, M.D.
April 15, 1998

Dr. Thomas E. Starzl, to my thinking, is the surgeon of this century. Holding fast to original thinking, willing to persist in what he believes right despite overwhelming majority objection, Tom's contributions are irrevocably imprinted on medicine. Barry and I cherished our association with Tom who though about the same age we regarded as our intellectual and moral father. Of physicians important to Barry, Starzl's name ranks at the very top.

Barry

Greatness, which comes in many guises, may be judged afterwards by a painting, book, musical composition or discovery that reveals nothing of the human price exacted for its production. Greatness also can be defined by the construction of a full and useful life under circumstances that would destroy most people. This was the way of Mildred (Barry) Friedman. It ennobled her, and it elevated everyone whom she touched.

Imagine the contrasting scenarios of the two parts of Barry's stay on earth. The first half was that of the charming, intelligent, and committed modern woman. She was a teacher, the idealistic wife of a remarkably committed physician, and the mother of three talented daughters. Then, in 1968, came the first of a series of hammer blows: the death of a premature fourth child, diabetes mellitus, adrenal insufficiency, cardiovascular-pulmonary disorders, blindness, and all of the complications of renal failure and its treatment with dialysis and kidney transplantation.

These disasters slowly crippled Barry physically, but never in spirit. Rather than yielding to her diseases, she tried first to learn from them, and then to disseminate her knowledge to help others. Although imprisoned by circumstances, she refused to be pathetic, and instead became a grand and highly functional inspiration. Her partner always was Eli, who ran the terrible gauntlet with her for 30 years. As the blows rained down, she never lowered her head or cried out for mercy. As a girl, Barry aspired to be a poet, and as a woman to be a writer. In the slender package she has left us, there is evidence that she succeeded in both objectives. How often does one find in a few sentences, or even in a phrase, so much meaning as can be found in her writings. These have been gathered here by Eli, not only to fill in the details of Barry s larger than life portrait, but because of their wealth of feeling and wisdom.

Thomas E. Starzl, M.D., Ph.D.
March 1, 1998

PREFACE

Having kidney failure is not a unique experience. Neither is receiving a kidney transplant or undergoing dialysis. Adopting to irreversible uremia — a devastating illness— by assisting others to cope with their own life trial represents the best of human traits. Bonded by marriage for 42 years, I was privileged to love and live with a marvelous and unique individual whose approach to life with this horrific disease taught me to regard every moment of our existence as precious. Preparation of this volume had two main objectives: 1) To honor the author for all of efforts in behalf of kidney patients. 2) To disseminate her insights and wisdom to those who may derive comfort and benefit from her words.

Mildred (Barry) Friedman was a medical writer and patient advocate devoted to the American Association of Kidney Patients, who died at University Hospital of Brooklyn on September 21st 1997 at the age of 61 of complications of type 1 diabetes. Barry, the second child of Leontine and Hardinge Barrett-Lennard, was born on October 17, 1935 in Manhattan and attended Brooklyn College as a New York State Scholarship Awardee earning a Bachelor of Arts degree in 1953. She subsequently began teaching in the New York City elementary schools gaining a Master's degree in education. Following the birth of her third child, Barry developed both diabetes and Addison's disease forcing her retirement from teaching.

Despite severe eye and kidney complications of diabetic vascular disease, Barry began a second career as an author of short stories and patient advice columns in publications of the American Association of Kidney Patients. In 1981, Barry developed kidney failure but after months of dialysis therapy underwent the then experimental treatment in diabetic patients of kidney transplantation with her sister Joan Hubbard as the donor. She regularly proffered straightforward coping recommendations in a section entitled Diabetic Directions. In 1992 she wrote: "By the time you read this my kidney and I will have celebrated our eleventh birthday. There is great joy in life even with all the complications of diabetes, even with feeling that I very well might have died eleven years ago and that at times I want to die now. My three girls have grown up, finished their educations, entered into good careers, met and then married the men they love, giving me the three great sons I never naturally had, and presented me with four (going on five) grandchildren. Seeing and holding and hugging and communicating with the next generation was something I never expected to experience."

Although progressive complications of diabetes including cardiac and cerebrovascular disease continued to necessitate intermittent hospitalizations, Barry made it a point to note that travel as far as the North Pole on a Russian Ice Breaker and most recently to Australia to visit relatives need not be omitted due to disability that sometimes mandated a wheelchair. Ten years following her kidney transplant, Mrs. Friedman invited her medical and professional associates and friends to a celebration at Windows On the World for which a musical show entitled "I'm Still Here" was written by Dennis Markell and Doug Cohen in which Ellen Foley and Ilene Kristen recounted highlights of her life. On the fifteenth anniversary of her transplant in February 1996, Barry chartered a boat for a dinner cruise around New York harbor again hosting a show called "Barry's Love Boat", starring Tovah Feldshuh. As cofounder and past president of the Diabetic Kidney Transplant Self-Help Group, a patient organization centered at University Hospital of Brooklyn where her transplant was performed, Barry promoted maximized activity and rehabilitation by often invalidated sufferers of multiple disorders attributed to diabetes. To ease the often-lengthy ordeal of clinic visits, Barry introduced and personally staffed a free beverage and literature cart for kidney patients. Barry was invited to share her positive approach to medical adversity by organ transplant and patient societies in Europe and throughout the United States. In her last unpublished column in which Barry described the experience of undergoing amputation of a toe while under local anesthesia, she remarked that "I'm still optimistic." Barry is survived by her husband Eli A. Friedman, a professor of medicine at SUNY, Health Science Center in Brooklyn and three daughters, Amy L. Friedman Meguira, a transplant surgeon at Yale, Rebecca Caspi a Foundation Administrator in Jerusalem Israel, and Sara Jo Grethlein a hematologist and Oncologist at SUNY, Health Science Center at Syracuse and seven grandchildren.

Other than the intensity of our love and the warm afterglow of our joyful years together, what I think of most in recalling who Barry was and how much she meant to me is that I can't think of a single instance when she wanted to harm anyone. Barry lacked the negative qualities of spitefulness, vindictiveness, and scheming. Indeed, her daily routine behavior standard became the epitome of what I strived to be but never quite attained. Now, read her words, chuckle over her gentle humor, and learn how precious the human spirit and will to live can be.

Eli A. Friedman
February 28, 1998

Table of Contents

COLUMNS

The Diabetic Foot 3
Eating 9
We Are All What We Eat 14
Pills Pills Pills 18
Survivors 21
Diabetic Directions: Travel Tricks and Advice 25
Medical Ethics 30
Diabetic Directions: Type 40
Holidays 44
Always Something New 49
Depressing Diabetes 56
DCCT — Bad or Good 62
...KneeBone Connected to the Thigh Bone, Thigh Bone Connected to the Hip Bone... 68
The Physical Side of Diabetes 74
The "L" Words. Liver, Lungs, Lymphatics 80
Skin 84
More About Diabetic Skin 90
Predictions 96
Sugar — Too Much, Too Little 100
I'm Trying To Think! 107

SHORT STORIES

The Attacker and the Waitress 116
Forgive Me Jack. Love Pop 123
Maiya's Daughter 131
Subway 143
A Funeral 150
Ma 156

Not Lucky 172
A Once Quiet Road 177

LETTERS AND COMMENTARY

Insulin Bottles 182
On Going Blind 191
On Being a Human Pincushion 195
Strange Heritage for an American 198
No Miracles 202
Tell Us Who You Are 204
Why? 208
Thanks Adrian 211
Ode to Willem Kolff 214
A New What? 216
Ruthie 219
My Husband 220

Columns

Barry, in 1989, recognized the ominous risk to lower limbs imparted by the triple threat of neuropathy, macrovasculopathy, and microvasculopathy. Warning about the danger imposed by foot disease in diabetic individuals, Barry presciently anticipated the complication that was to end her life: "When things progress to amputation it is not only sad, but life threatening." Being aware of the complications of diabetes may not protect the individual from a duration related and perhaps inescapable risk. Nevertheless, the informed diabetic patient may be able to delay, minimize, and even avoid loss of limbs. Based on Barry's concern and protective effort, our Renal Clinic has had a participating podiatrist for twenty years. Following a toe fracture in a non-feeling foot, a non-healing ulcer, despite repetitive vascular bypass attempts .induced systemic infection that terminated Barry's struggle against an inexorable disease.

The Diabetic Foot.

Self help groups can have an effect on diabetic feet. I'll tell you 2 stories which happened while I was acting as a member of our group. A blind diabetic woman who, over the course of several years had had some serious problems with her feet, was busy telling me how she hated the way oxfords looked. I gave her a couple of suggestions: wear the same color stocking as shoe - it makes them stand out less, and in the winter wear flat, round toe boots with socks - no-one would know the difference. The suggestions worked. Second story: while visiting transplant patients in the hospital, I saw a lovely young blind girl being walked along the corridor BAREFOOT. Never having met her before I still had the nerve to tell her that she had no control over losing her sight or her kidneys but that she darn well could try to keep herself from losing legs. Next time I saw her, she was wearing slippers. What did I mean by my statement? About 25% of diabetics will develop foot problems related to their disease and 20% of all diabetic hospital admissions are for foot problems. Also between one half and two thirds of the lower limb amputations performed in the U.S. are done on diabetics.

According to Rausher, Rausher, and Friedman working in Brooklyn, 50% of these amputations can be avoided. Of the foot problems that lead to surgery, 92.5% are preventable. Their study showed 42.5% of the foot problems were due to wearing the wrong shoes, 12.5% due to walking barefoot at night (usually to go to the toilet), and 35% were self-inflicted (soaking, chemical corn and callus removers, scratching, etc.). Diabetics are more prone to pedal disease conditions because of neuropathy and poor circulation. They may or may not be more apt to have infections than normal people but when infections occur they progress more rapidly.

Neuropathy, a loss of sensation, can lead to ignoring wounds or bad fitting shoes. Cuts, calluses, or breaks in the skin must be treated. Thick corns and calluses should be treated by a podiatrist. Calluses can be thick enough to act as pebbles caught in shoes. Because these conditions can't be felt, daily visual inspections of diabetic feet must be carried out. If the patient has trouble seeing, or can't bend enough, a second person should be involved. The same reasoning applies to forbidding diabetics to cut their own nails, calluses, or corns. Not everybody must go to a professional for this type of care. Files can be used so no damage to normal skin occurs.

Neuropathy can affect weight bearing. Normally the foot senses where the greatest pressure is being applied and shifts slightly so as to spread that pressure over greater surfaces. In the diabetic, pressure can continue to be present in one spot causing ulceration through a process known as progressive autolysis. There is a fine balance between toe extenders and toe flexors to distribute weight during walking. After healing an ulcer, it is important to know the cause of the lesion because 83% of those who returned to the same shoes had a recurrence in the same spot, while only 26% with special shoes did. Levin of Washington University in St. Louis, whose statistics these are, even suggests such radical things as job changes to avoid the kind of foot use in the old job.

As a side effect of neuropathy, it can lead to the purchase of poorly fitting shoes. With the loss of sensation, diabetics tend to buy tighter and tighter shoes so they can "feel" them.

When the neuropathy is of the peripheral motor kind it can lead to a loss of muscular tone and atrophy which allows the small bones of the foot to shift and cause deformities such as bunions. When some muscles are weaker than others claw or hammer toes can be the result and these often have attendant ulcers on the knuckles.

Poor circulation is another complication of diabetes. Peripheral vascular disease can lead to hardening of the arteries due to calcium, cholesterol, lipid, and platelet deposition with migration of smooth muscle cells into the lumen of the vessels. This narrows the channels so oxygen, nutrients, and antibiotics can't get to where they are needed. If oxygen and food don't get to an area, tissue may start to die. Clots further complicate the supply problem keeping white blood cells, which fight infection, away as well. Two other factors tangle the situation: 1. diabetics deposit calcium in blood vessels making them hard and 2. diabetics don't find new blood routes as easily as normal people do. Symptoms of poor circulation include: pain in the legs when walking fast or uphill, leg pain while lying down, a red or purple foot when the foot is dangled, loss of hair from feet or toes, dry and shiny skin on the foot, and a white fungus under the toenails. Clogged arteries can be scrapped clean, opened with a balloon technique, or surgically bypassed.

Nontreatable risk factors include heredity, age and duration of diabetes. Controllable factors are smoking, blood pressure, blood sugar and lowering of cholesterol and triglycerides. In order to improve the circulation patients must stop smoking, lower their cholesterol, exercise, and reduce their weight.

When neuropathy and poor circulation lead to ulceration, infection is a common occurrence. Infection is bad in diabetics for several reasons. It can lead to high blood sugars which are detrimental in themselves and have a harmful side effect. Neutrophils, the attacking white blood cells, are weakened by high glucose levels and don't engulf organisms according to George Eisenbarth of the Joslyn Clinic. McIntyre of Arizona, reports that with good sugar control phagocytosis improves but not to the same degree as in normals.

Infected diabetic foot ulcers show all kinds of organisms - gram positive and gram negative, cocci and bacilli, aerobes and anaerobes. Cultures should be taken deep in the wound and not superficially. There are occasional pure cultures usually Staph aureus. Fierer, Daniel, and Davis have data that shows of 30 diabetics with lower extremity infections that required surgical intervention, 17 had mixed aerobes and anaerobes, and 6 had Staph aureus alone (these patients did better than the other group). Conditions like these call for treatment with a broad spectrum antibiotic aimed at aerobes and anaerobes, debridement (dead tissue is an excellent culture medium) and total bed rest. Three things about bed rest: weight bearing on an infected ulcer can cause the pus to spread into the planar areas of the foot, diabetics who try to walk avoiding pressure on the area often can't because they don't feel when they are stepping on it, and it is difficult to get compliance at home because there is no pain. A process called contact casting can be used on selected patients. Contact casts differ from fracture casts in that they have no lining and are molded directly to the foot to avoid friction. They must be changed after 3-5 days to take a loss of edema into account.

When things progress to amputation it is not only sad, but life threatening. Loss of limbs is 15 times more likely in diabetics than in nondiabetics. Levin at Washington University in St. Louis also states that diabetic inhospital mortality is 3%, that 35% do not survive 3 years, and 59% do not survive for 5 years. That is a high rate of mortality. Moreover, 42% will lose the other leg within 1-3 years, and 56% in 3-5 years because the same pathological processes are present and the remaining leg has to deal with increased pressure and work load. Each amputation costs about $30,000 without taking into account the prosthesis, job loss, disability payments, and changes in the quality of life. Good blood sugar control is important here as well because two groups (Cruse and Foord and Verta) state that poorly controlled diabetics have higher incidences of wound infection but that well controlled patients may heal as well as patients without diabetes.

Let us now get into some of the causes of neuropathy and poor circulation. It is known that diabetics have increased blood viscosity. A red blood cell measures 7.4 microns, white cells are slightly larger and the lumen of the capillaries is 3-5 microns. Therefore the circulating cells must deform to fit through the capillaries and in diabetics some of this flexibility is lost. A medication, pentoxifylline (Trental) improves the pliability of red and white blood cells but takes weeks or months to work. Therefore, it has no applicability for acute lesions. Thickening of capillary basement membranes (a finding in diabetics) may make diffusion of nutrients through the wall difficult and make leukocyte entrance into areas of infection hard. Nonenzymatic glycosylation of collagen and proteoglycans alters the molecular substructure of basement membranes which may lead to altered secretions of basement membrane compounds. The formation of heparin sulfate which has to do with the anionic filtration barrier, may be interfered with. The sorbitol pathway is also of consequence in peripheral neuropathy since the increase in sorbitol causes a decrease in myoinositol which is essential for nerve function. Control of blood sugar should minimize the effects of glycosylation and sorbitol formation.

Easier to affect, and just as necessary, is the wearing of proper shoes. Remember the Rausher data that 42.5% of foot lesions were due to poor footgear. By law, slaves were not allowed to wear shoes in ancient Egypt but other people did. Sandals and moccasins are the basic styles and all other fashions are a combination of these. It wasn't until the 19th century that rights were made different from lefts. In early America, an itinerant shoemaker lived with a family long enough to make a year's supply for each member of the group, and then moved on. The elevated shoes and heels worn by women in ancient times, disappeared until the middle ages when Louis XV demanded them because he was short. You should know that feet change with the season, daily temperature, time of day, sitting, standing, or lying, age, and changes in weight. Dynamic forces on the sole are the most important factors in correcting faulty areas of pressure. These can be recorded with infrared thermography, or footprints in special microcapsule socks. When it comes to fitting shoes, comfort is most important. Sellers should look at old shoes to see where they have lost their shape due to pressure. Space should be left in front of the big toe and the other toes should not be compressed sideways. As an aside, physicians should know of neighborhood stores with knowledgeable fitters.

Good shoes are a significant element in proper diabetic care and so should education of patients to the daily foot inspection. Because diabetic feet are so prone to unnoticed problems, attention must be paid to them daily. Patients should be instructed to inspect their feet in the same light and position. They should know the color of their skin and the shape of their feet. Calluses, corns, blisters, and breaks in the skin are noted while keeping in mind that infected areas may feel firmer. Persistent, unpleasant odors are meaningful. Feet should be lotioned with noncosmetic preparations (alcohol dries) after bathing but not between the toes. Caution should be expressed over the use of hot water bottles, bare feet, home surgery of corns and calluses, soaking feet, and using band-aids. Recommendations are made that diabetics change their shoes at least once a day and that they exercise (walking is best). Choice of shoes should be made clear by physicians or podiatrists.

Round toe, flat, leather, oxfords are the acceptable style although nowadays with fashion allowing the use of sneakers or running shoes that is also satisfactory. Doctors' checking of shoes and feet of diabetics is necessary for good care.

Patient education is pressing but so is physician education. In a clinic, Levin found that only 12-16% of diabetic feet were examined. That is deplorable. Shoes and socks should be removed during every medical visit.

Modern medical care options often lead to feelings of despondency because situations cannot be cured. Here is a situation which can be kept from occurring in over 90% of the cases. Amputations can be avoided. Moreover, the ability to ambulate comfortably contributes to the success of all therapeutic regimens.

Without question, a key stress for Barry and others with insulin treated diabetes is construction of sensible meals according to what has been termed a diabetic diet. For those with renal failure, the complexities are compounded by the need to restrict protein and phosphorous. Barry was working on a Renal Diet Book when she died. This 1996 column gives some of her thoughts.

EATING

Normal human beings eat. Nonnormal human beings eat too. Most people consume what they want, when they want, if they want. Not so for diabetics and the situation worsens for diabetics who use the artificial kidney to stay alive. The renal-diabetic diet is complicated and confining.

Fifteen and a half years ago when dialysis started for me, I was handed a renal diet sheet and told to meld it with my diabetic diet. There were problems galore. At that time, patients were allowed to become much sicker before renal replacement therapy was begun, than they are today. With increasing uremia there is decreasing mental ability. My mind wasn't functioning. Adding to my dilemma were the terms in which the renal diet was written. Yes, exchange units were noted. (Exchanges are a way of giving portion sizes for food so that you can keep track of what and how much you are eating.) Diabetic exchange lists, published jointly by both ADAs: American Diabetic Association and American Dietetic Association, give the parameters for one exchange in each category. Carbohydrate, protein, dairy, vegetable, fruit, and fat are the classifications. My new renal list had some things measured for 3 exchanges, some for 1. If my personal diet prescription called for 2 exchanges and the renal list had that particular kind of food as 3 exchanges, I was lost. It was a short fight. Dialysis only lasted for a few months and then my sister donated a kidney. Shortly thereafter, my brain was working again. The "Renal Diabetic Diet" which is still used in many institutions, was the result. Foods were listed in terms of one exchange thus simplifying the math needed to fill an individual diet order. Of course it was checked for accuracy by experts.

Now let's step back a bit and talk about food and diabetes. Nourishment is not only a necessity for diabetics, it is also a medicine. Blood sugar and therefore, the disease, is controlled by a complicated mix of antihyperglycemic drugs (insulin or orals), exercise and food. Pharmaceuticals given to keep blood sugar levels within the normal bounds, are timed. I will talk about insulin because I know it best. There are various kinds of insulin. Their timings differ. Some begin quickly. Some, after many hours. Some have a long lasting effect. Some, shorter. Patients know what they take and when the action begins and when it peaks. A blood sugar level is determined by sticking a finger, getting a drop of blood, putting that on a chemically treated strip, waiting about a minute, and reading a value with the help of a meter. Size of insulin dose is determined and administered and then, about 30 minutes later, the patient gets to eat.

But what can that person eat? Along with drug prescriptions, a diet prescription is handed out. Just as an example here's mine: Breakfast - 1 carbohydrate, 1 fat, and ½ dairy exchange. Lunch - 2 vegetable, 1 fruit, 2 carbohydrate. Dinner - 3 lean meat exchanges, 2 vegetable, 1 fruit, 2 carbohydrate exchanges. Snack - 1 carbohydrate, 1 protein exchange. Sounds simple but I have yet to figure a way to margarine my Cheerios for breakfast! Official exchange lists tell me portion sizes. Mixing foods within a list is fine. Go ahead and spread peanut butter on your shrimp if you want but remember to measure the quantity you use.

OK. Now I have kinds of food and portion sizes but I also have to pay attention to the times for my meals. Eating at approximately the same hour each day is the best way to go. Using a schedule helps keep my insulin doses overlapping correctly so that I always have insulin coverage. Smooth sailing should lie ahead but here come the waves. High waves.

Kidney failure is here. You need dialysis. With dialysis comes the renal diet. Diabetes is still present and you must account for type and portion of what you put in your mouth but now you have to calculate the sodium, potassium, phosphorus, and fluid in what you consume. Certain things are put on a "NO NO" list. Citrus fruits, bananas, and more than just a little tomato, as well as liquids, are forbidden. I felt that all good things to eat had been taken away from me. Maybe 3 foods were left and all were broiled or boiled and none were interesting. Did you feel that way? But that isn't true. Good meals lie ahead.

I have procrastinated. I have been lazy but the time has come. A cookbook for diabetics on hemodialysis is in the works. Friends are helping me test the recipes. So far they are enjoying the dishes they prepare. Nutritional or dietetic training are not in my past but I bring some mathematical skills for figuring out nutritional content per portion and the ability to read lists. I am sure I will make some mistakes but I do believe my analysis will be in the right ball park.

Vegetables were chosen as the first work area because they are the most difficult for dialysis patients. Renal diets limit potassium content to 2000 mg. per day and veggies can be high in potassium. A single portion is ½ cup. Some low potassium vegetables (up to 125 mg.) are: cabbage, frozen cauliflower, frozen carrots, and leeks. Note that a few are cooked from *frozen.* Brussel sprouts, all kidney, lima, pinto, etc. beans, spinach, potatoes, and tomatoes are part of the group containing over 250 mg. potassium. Sounds pretty bad doesn't it? but wait ... here is the smiley part. It is probably your only chance to dialyze something besides yourself. Potatoes, peeled and cut into whatever shape you want and any other vegetable that is solid, like parsnips, can be soaked in a large quantity of water overnight, drained, rinsed and cooked as you wish. Dialyzing them like this cuts the potassium content by half.

Dairy products contain high potassium levels as do bananas, raisins, and melons. Most carbohydrates are safe to consume.

Stay away from canned produce, because it frequently contains large amounts of sodium. Making food tasty can be accomplished. Put together a small collection of dried herbs. Include oregano, thyme, basil, dill, curry, cumin, and pepper. You will like some better than others. At the right time of year, many of these can be found fresh in the market. Fresh is always best. Remember to use more of the fresh than of the dried. Stay away from anything with "salt" in its name like garlic salt, celery salt, etc.

Caution should be taken with salt substitutes because most of them are high in potassium. Pepper does a pretty good job of disguising the lack of salt. Use nonstick cookware to reduce the amount of oil needed for sauteing. I find I can fry a zillion pounds of onion in 1 tsp. oil. Olive oil is a good choice.

Following a restrictive diet, understanding what is in the dishes you eat, staying away from the "No No's" requires that you cook. Food preparation can take a lot of clicks of the clock. Some people like kitchen time. Some don't. There are ways around the dilemma. Cook large quantities, divide it into correct portions and freeze in correct size containers. Voila! You have created your own frozen dinners. You might also opt to eat the same thing for a week or however long it takes you to finish what you made. Strange as it sounds, I prefer this choice. I won't want to look at that stuff again for a long time but I do enjoy the consumption. Each to her own. Different strokes for different folks. I seldom claim to be normal.

Speaking of normal, my cookbook will look strange to the average person. Soups are not included. After all, they are fluid and you are very limited in your fluid intake. There will also not be many deserts. We are diabetics and are told to stay away from sweet things. Even with the current liberation of dietary definitions, we must control how much sugar we eat. Have you seen the new (June 1995) lists? Simple sugars (table sugar, doughnuts) and complex carbohydrates (pasta, potatoes, corn) are now considered to convert to the same glucose in the body and are therefore interchangeable. Yes, you can eat pie, cookies, cake guilt free. Don't add these things to what you eat but substitute for the complex carbohydrates in your diet. Nobody is saying "have a large piece of chocolate cake every day." but some, once in a while, is fine. I like the new "free" list which adds a few things. A bit of ketchup on *whatever* tastes good. Take caution. I was advised that while blood sugar can be kept under good control when you eat this way, triglycerides may rise. Watch and see what happens to you and then adjust.

Maybe, by this time, you are understanding my approach to food. We face the activity of eating at least three times a day. Food consumption is necessary to stay alive. Quality of life is important. Enough control over this part of my life is given to me so that pleasure can result. I stay middle of the road in most things. I follow the diabetic diet restrictions most of the time but when the urge to cheat builds up - I cheat. Keeping track of the times I don't follow my regimen becomes a new activity. When I was on dialysis sage advice was given me by a physician who, himself, had been on dialysis for many years. "Cheat the night before treatment." Makes sense.

In this column published in Nephrology News & Issues in February 1995, pgs.22-24, Barry explains the drill demanded of insulin treated diabetics. As she puts it: "What do I have to do to try to avoid a second go-round with renal failure? Compliance is very necessary and so is cheating. If a diet, any diet, becomes unpleasant and unsatisfying, out the window it goes. Guilt is not allowed; neither is self-indulgence. Many years have gone by and now I find myself suffering from burnout."

We Are All What We Eat

...but more so if we are diabetics. I am amused when people say: "It's such a good healthy diet." It is exactly that but compliance is not a simple matter. At first, after my diagnosis, because I felt no different if I stuck to my diet or not, my food consumption changed little. Sugary edibles remained part of my fare. Frequency of consuming simple carbohydrates dropped and I did try to put my prescribed proportions of the five food groups into practice. Portion sizes were not accurately gauged. When, fifteen years later, diabetic complications muddled my life, the realization that diabetes is a lousy disease and that I should control my diet, hit home. Like drinking for a reformed drunk, compliance became very important. If I can protect my kidney transplant from diabetic nephropathy, I will. Fourteen years later it is still doing well but the future may hold a different prognosis.

What do I have to do to try to avoid a second go-round with renal failure?

As a Type I (insulin dependent) diabetic, I never just eat. Thirty years ago when my diagnosis was made, the exchange system for measuring food portions, was explained to me. The concept of food exchanges allows whoever uses it, to vary meal content while maintaining a standard intake of the major food groups.

Let me start again. There are five exchange lists: protein, carbohydrate, fat, dairy, and fruit and vegetable. Doctors prescribe specific eating patterns for each patient. I am allowed ½ milk exchange, 1 carbohydrate exchange, and 1 fat exchange for breakfast.

If I look at the American Diabetes Association carbohydrate exchange list, my choice for 1 exchange is 3/4 cup dry cereal, ½ English muffin, 1 slice of bread, ½ bagel (little bagels - not the huge New York ones), etc.. These portions are all equal in calories, amount of fat, amount of protein, and amount of dairy products. Therefore, I can choose any one of them. My usual morning meal is dry cereal because it satisfies me. I have not, however, figured out how to butter Cheerios. (Common sense is necessary so my one fat exchange is ignored. Patients can combine strange food choices as long as they use the correct (for them) number of exchanges. My very favorite sandwich includes peanut butter, bologna, and cheese. One ounce of each provides me with the three protein exchanges I get for supper. "Yuck" you say but note I haven't invited you for dinner. Variety is, for me, an important way of keeping on my diet and compliance is necessary. I like to cook so regulating meals is really at my discretion.

Type I diabetes is treated with diet, insulin, and exercise. Food then, becomes a medicine. Attempting to balance providing glucose from edibles and using glucose through metabolism, complicates life. Because I take two insulins, NPH (an intermediate acting insulin - works for up to 16 hours) and Regular (short acting - about a 4 hour duration), the doses of these drugs must be administered at approximately the same time each day. Insulin is injected thirty minutes before a meal providing peak action as food is absorbed, so my meals should be at approximately the same time each day. If this isn't done, occasionally too much insulin will be in the bloodstream and at other moments, too little. Too much insulin leads to a low blood sugar which is always an emergency requiring immediate correction. Too little insulin causes high blood sugar levels and can result in ketoacidosis and coma. I'm lucky. My family and friends understand. They pleasantly bend to me and eat according to my schedule. Not everyone has such cooperation.

Content, portion size, and timing are all important but what happens when things are different? The invitation comes. An affair has been arranged. I want to go but they plan to feed me at 9 o'clock at night or in the middle of the afternoon or for brunch. I've played with many possible solutions. None works. When dinner will be late, I take my NPH at the regular time (6 o'clock) and the regular half an hour before I *think* I will be served. Midafternoon repasts are dealt with by checking my blood sugar at my usual lunch time and if it's OK, I wait until thirty minutes before I *think* I will be presented with food and take extra regular insulin because I know I'm going to eat more than my usual small lunch. However, the question now is: What to do for supper? Well, hungry or not, at the usual hour I take my insulin but less regular, because I'm not about to eat what I normally do. Notice please that I said I take insulin thirty minutes before I *think* food will appear. Asking a waiter or waitress when this will occur gives me a probable time schedule. Other problems exist. Brunch is not easy. Sleeping late is out. If I get up, take insulin, and eat I can go back to bed but somehow it aint the same.

Sick days, hungry days present other quandaries. I don't go to bed early because I must eat my evening snack. If I don't feel like eating, or can't, I take less regular insulin, eat what I can, and check blood sugar levels with finger sticks, more often. Being hungry is easier to deal with now that the artificial sweeteners lower the calorie count in many items on the supermarket shelves. Raw vegetables work but I find I tire of them. Pickles are good but how many pickles can you eat? Diet soda works to fill me up as do low calorie ice pops or fudgicles. My latest solution is the new to the market, sugar free JELL-O cups (in your dairy case) which are FREE at only 10 calories a serving.

Restaurants raise questions. Like most people, I have certain establishments to which I return. My family laughs at me. When I'm going to eatery #1, I don't have to study the menu. I did that years ago and know what they offer that fits my diet and that I enjoy. For eatery #2 I use the same approach. When the restaurant is new to me, I peruse the card trying to fit what I require to what is proffered. I also ask questions. Is this prepared with sugar? Is your fresh fruit salad really fresh or did some of it come out of a can? Explaining the reason for questioning isn't necessary. Restaurants are now accustomed to people with special requirements.

Airplanes can be difficult. Hospitals aren't the easiest places either. I always provide for myself. I look at what's in front of me and chose what to eat. Meals for diabetics are not ordered in the air (yes in the hospital) because I do not want someone else to judge my portion sizes and proportions of the five food groups. My carry-on always holds stuff I can eat. If I haven't gotten enough or if I'm stuck someplace without a meal, or if the dietician forgot to send up my evening snack, packaged cheese or peanut butter and crackers as well as little boxes of raisins calm my fears and yes, I do worry about where my next meal is coming from.

Foreign countries present me with a real dilemma. If I can, I choose to eat American style but if I can't, I eat what's on my plate and hope. Staying home because food compliance is not possible is not my cup of tea. I do ask if things such as fruit juices have been sweetened and avoid those that have. This is in complete accord with my philosophy that I am a person with a disease, not a disease with legs.

Exchange lists are not the only way to measure food. It is the system first introduced to me. I work with it easily and after all these years food rationing is automatic. Occasionally, I truly use measuring cups, spoons and scales but most often I just eyeball what I eat.

Compliance is very necessary and so is cheating. If a diet, any diet, becomes unpleasant and unsatisfying, out the window it goes. Seldom do I consume sweets but if I really want something, I eat it. Guilt is not allowed; neither is self-indulgence. Many years have gone by and now I find myself suffering from burnout. Recognizing the circumstance, I've eased up a bit. Time will settle me back in my routine and I'm not allowing myself to get out of control, but last week's ice cream cone tasted good.

As a professional patient, Barry was a keen observer of people. Barry noted other patients consulting their pharmacists on a multitude of problems. Repeatedly, Barry referred relatives to their pharmacists for ideas on how to travel with medications that require refrigeration or other special handling. People who deal daily with a large number of pills have their own dilemmas. In this 1994 column Barry recounts her own coping mechanisms.

Pills Pills Pills

and more pills. These days I take 25 pills, caplets, tablets, capsules or whatever you want to call them, every 24 hours. The number has been higher and even, once, lower. It is the way I remember how to count. Other positive forces result - like game playing.

Smirking is one of my favorite little games and I smirk happily when I overhear someone say: "Oh, I hate to take a pill." So do I but I swallow them by the handful. There are little amusements. Shall I take the three big ones and then all the little ones? How about approximately equal group sizes? What colors go together? Does a long flat one followed by a small circular one make an exclamation mark and will my stomach understand what I am trying to say? How is my color vision loss today? Yup. There's the blue one and the dark green and white is easy but what are these guys - white, tan, pink, or yellow? Oh boy - a simple to identify specimen. Looks like two round ones stuck together. That's just the morning set.

Dinner and bed time call for more.

Let's see - there are the timed ones - breakfast and supper consumption will take care of them but wait a minute. Here's a big flat circular one that has to be taken two at a time, half an hour before breakfast and supper. I guess I can remember those.

Success was mine when I convinced the doctors to clot them all into just three groups. I refused to schedule myself for midmorning or midafternoon doses. They'd be forgotten. It doesn't sound like it but I do do things besides take medicines and when I'm involved in other projects, I'm involved - not a patient. My disease or diseases must learn to live with ME not me with them. Easy to say but I'm human. I do get depressed, maddened at what has happened to me. Nobody wanted to grow up handicapped, trapped in a body that doesn't work very well. I've come to the conclusion that my body is lucky I still talk to it. But there are good things to keep me going.

As I pill pop, it occurs to me that I'm glad my pills have minds of their own. What do you mean? You don't think they have minds? OK. Please explain to me, how do they know where to go? When I swallow 10 of 'em, they seem to get where they belong. One doesn't just follow another and arrive in the wrong spot. They get where they belong. No minds? HAH

Pills have more marvelous properties. Mine like to travel. I know because they eagerly jump into my little sandwich bags when I announce a trip is coming up. My tricks for globe wandering with them are simple. Well, maybe not simple but they work. First, I make two sets of drugs - one for my purse, one for my suitcase. That way if one is lost or stolen, drowned or burned, I'm not out of business. They're always right with me. I won't let happen to me what happened to a man I know. Caught in the big San Francisco earthquake, he added his own set of shudders to the movement of the pavement when he realized his Cyclosporine was 15 floors up in a hotel whose elevators were now electricity free. So he climbed and climbed and climbed. Not me. I'm lazy.

Anyhow, back to my globe-trotting medicines. Days before the trip, I bring all my bottles to the kitchen table, add a pile of plastic sandwich bags and a cup of coffee to keep me alert. Let's say it's a 10 day trip ahead of me. Twelve sandwich bags are arranged on the table (have you ever tried to get sandwich bags to sit on a surface - open?). In order, the correct number of each kind of pill is dropped into each bag and the top knotted. I can hear you. You're saying: "Why 12 for a 10 day trip?" I'm as nutty as anybody. The extra 2 are for a short highjacking. Back to my little plastic bags. The next one contains 12 sets of dinner-time pills. They're easy to tell apart - one kind is big and the other small. Tie up the bag and on to bedtime potions. Different colors and sizes so they can go into the same container - 12 sets and tie a knot. Next come the emergency supplies, once in a while stuff including antibiotics and pain killers - into a bag, knot at the top. Finally all the little bags go into the master bag which is usually too full to knot at the top. Rubber band to the rescue. Another cup of coffee. Another set of pills and my major packing is done. Clothes? 5 minutes - no more.

When the trip is shorter, like to a restaurant for dinner, pill packing is less complicated. I'm beginning to acquire a selection of little pill boxes. Speaking of pill boxes, think for a minute of the pill organizers you have seen advertised. I admire them and turn away. Not big enough spaces for my morning collection, not the right compartments, too large to carry but pretty colors, pretty colors. Anyway, time to get ready for dinner out. Pill box selected, I bring out the pill bottles. Always prepared, I decide to put in enough for 2 restaurant excursions. That involves putting in one extra of the little orange guys which I frequently manage to drop on restaurant floors. They're important, don't skip ones, so I try to plan for my clumsiness. So far, it works.

Last but not least, let me tell you the story of Charlie, my goldfish. At home, at suppertime, I take my pills and then feed Charlie. It's a way of not forgetting him. But the day came when I dropped a pill into Charlie's aquarium. Strong medicine. Instant aquarium cleaning. Love that fish. Won't share my pills with him!

If any single article epitomized Barry's philosophy, this is it. During a trip to the Catskill Mountains with family, Barry attended a performance by Ben Vereen in which he sang, joked, and actually danced in a wheelchair. The experience evoked one of Barry's last columns for AAKP in 1996.

Survivors

I've seen a wheelchair dancing. Dancing magnificently. Dancing as part of Ben Vereen. As I watched the performance the performer won my respect and admiration. I honor and acclaim survivors and this man fits the bill. A while ago he was almost totaled in an accident. Nobody expected him to walk again. He walked. He walked earlier than anyone thought he would. He danced.

Bodies, as we know, don't always do what we want them to and Ben Vereen's knees gave way. The reason could be dancing on them too soon or still the old accident or just a life-time of cavorting. I don't think it matters because the result was two knee replacements. New joints require their owner to allow them to heal. So patients have to stay off them and only gradually use them. Mr. Vereen, therefore, was in a wheelchair.

Now, I'm not a dancer or even an athlete but I know that certain people have total control of their body motions. For them, every little muscle movement is managed, not always consciously, but in an ordered way. Actions that work are natural and flow. Things that are contrived look that way. They look labored which can be either good or bad but Mr. Vereen's gestures came across to me as, simply, right. The wheelchair had become an extension of his body, an inherent part of his person. It never occurred to me that a wheelchair could dance but it can.

At the end of the show the dancer disappeared backstage. A few minutes later he reappeared and *walked* slowly to center stage using two canes. He won't be kept down. He manages. He copes. He is a survivor.

And you too, are survivors. Whether you are the patient who has lived through End Stage Renal Disease (Look at those words. They mean Fatal Kidney Failure.) or the loved one who lives next to it, you are survivors. Because you are reading this magazine, I know that you are intelligently involved with your disease, that you want to learn about it, that you want to go on.

ESRD is not a simple thing to live with. Good days and bad days happen. Medications have to be managed. You have to keep an eye on your supply and take them when you should. Appointments have to be made and kept. Diabetics must keep records and do unpleasant things to themselves like sticking fingers to do blood sugars and injecting themselves if they take insulin. Meals must be thought out and timed. Nasty episodes, like insulin reactions for those on insulin, must be treated immediately with the sugar source you have arranged to have with you. Dialysis patients must know where their next treatment will be or, for CAPD patients, that the supplies they require are at hand. That's the physical part.

The emotional part is more subtle. Even when with other patients a smile, a joke, a laugh characterize our survivors. Sure, we have complaints and problems but we deal with them. We may squeak a bit but then it's the squeaky wheel that gets the grease and sometimes we need grease. Look around you. Find out how many years that patient and this one have been on treatment. Called "chronic diseases" our illnesses don't get cured; don't go away. We learn to live with them and around them. I mean by that, that other aspects of our lives get much of our energy and concentration. We live.

Other survivors are probably better known than we are. I think of Franklin Delano Roosevelt who overcame the crippling effects of polio and rose to fill the highest position in the land. You may be an FDR fan or not but admiration for his successful efforts should be part of his image. During his presidency the world was a madhouse. War was declared. We fought on two fronts. He traveled to meet other world leaders. His medical problems (and they were more than just paralysis) were not in the news reports. He just went on.

Julio Iglesias was a professional soccer player. There was a car accident. "You will never walk again." the doctors said. Well, Mr. Iglesias crawled on the floor and learned to walk again but he needed another career. Good decision. Now as a rich singer, he is also a survivor. He didn't give up.

Without sight and without hearing, the child Helen Keller didn't give up either. Both senses were lost early in her life due to an illness but with the aid of a great companion, she entered the world and conquered it. She learned to speak, to listen with her hands, to physically write. She was grumpy at times. We're all allowed a grump or two. Books were written. Trips were taken. Friends were made. She coped. She survived.

Illness is not the only thing people overcome and survive. Stories in the newspapers tell of people who jumped over prejudice and did good things. Recently, an aged laundress made the news for giving her life savings (a considerable sum) to a university for scholarships. She had dropped out of school at the age of eight. She lived poor. Now the president has come to see her. She visits New York City and even wears high heels when she feels it is necessary. An honorary degree from Harvard is hers. A picture of her hangs at the university she benefited and it is the first picture of an African American ever to be displayed in those hallowed halls. We can only imagine what troubles she lived through. She is a survivor.

While in Denver for the AAKP convention, I went to the museum to see an exhibit on the Buffalo Soldiers. Buffalo Soldiers were black men who joined the army after the Civil War. They were not allowed into white units. Not allowed to command themselves. They were governed by white officers. The record these soldiers achieved was excellent. Good fighters in the field, they fought another battle. As slaves, they had been forbidden to read or write so, when they were in the army, classrooms were set up for them and they won that fight, too. I was impressed and couldn't get them out of my mind. Later, at the AAKP reception, I chose to sit at a table with a man who was alone. I told him of my afternoon. He looked at me with a quizzical expression on his face and said: "I am a Buffalo Soldier". We spoke and he told me of the black regiment he had been part of during the second World War. Again, these men were not deemed worthy to command themselves and their officers were white. Their record was extraordinary. Now this man had fatal kidney disease. He had lived with the prejudices of his time and now was dealing with his illness. He is a survivor and I was honored to have had a conversation with him.

People go on. The Pope and Mother Theresa do not ask for sympathy; they merely go back to work. Ben Vereen used a wheelchair and so did competitors in the Transplant Olympics. What a zest for life they have. I think we have all known others who have just given up and wait around to die. Some aid the process. But then there is a Christopher Reeve. Almost totally paralyzed from the neck down, he has resumed his career. Yes, I think he is still Superman and this time for real.

You are for real, too. Life is lived. Sure medical problems take a lot of time, yet I think you enjoy yourselves with an equal amount of energy. I've attended many AAKP conventions and talked to a lot of people. There was usually a laugh, a smile, a joke and a reaching out for the solution to a problem but seldom a complaint. It may be there. I've never heard it - the "Why me?" question.

As I meet you, or just know that you are out there, I am happy to be one of you, part of the group. However, my mind is busy telling me that we should have a theme song. How about "I'm Still There" or maybe "My Way"?

Traveling was an important component of Barry's activities. Comprehending the challenge imposed by trying to juggle insulin, time zones, activities, and meals can be overwhelming. Barry's "tricks and advice" imparted in this 1996 column have been helpful to many who employed them.

Diabetic Directions: Travel Tricks and Advice

What's in a name? Well, let's see. *Diabetic Directions*. North, South, East, West - I'm ready to go but then I'm a traveler. There are lots of places I haven't journeyed to yet but there are many I have. Just last summer I was 300 miles from the North Pole. African safaris, trains in Switzerland, the Hermitage, and "daughter visiting" in Israel have all been on the itinerary. My travel tricks and advice may not be the most expert but they help *me* wander in comparative comfort and with little worry.

As a first suggestion: Don't hide your illness, particularly if it is diabetes. There are times when you need help and you must always plan. As soon as I see a flight attendant on a plane, my mouth opens: "I an a diabetic and need to know when meals will be served so I can schedule my insulin."

Usually the answer is not only swift but accompanied by a : "Do you need anything now? Tell me when you do." And that's the end of it. If I act strangely, someone has a clue as to "Why?". I always wear my medical dog tag which identifies me as a diabetic with a kidney transplant and gives a phone number where my personal medical information is available.

Other people who should be told are traveling companions. "I'm hard to journey with. I need three meals a day and they have to be approximately on time." Luck is on my side. My friends pleasantly acquiesce but independence remains my goal.

Some things, such as planning mealtimes, require cooperation from others but for the most part I provide for myself. This does mean I carry a *large* purse. Besides what every woman carries there are my supply of pills for the journey plus some extras (enough to cover me during a short hijacking), sources of fast sugar (jelly beans for me), food in case I'm stuck some place without (ever sat in a plane for hours?), and my blood sugar kit which includes swabs, syringes, and two kinds of insulin sufficient for my voyage plus - you guessed it - some extras.

Speaking of insulin, I find my requirements shift when I am on the go. Perhaps extra activity or stress account for the changes but whatever does it, I am aware of the variation and raise or lower my dose as needed. Of course when you cross time zones there are predictable alterations. The size of short-acting insulin (Regular) doses depend on the meal and don't change. Amounts of intermediate-acting insulin (Lente or NPH) do vary because the doses overlap and you don't want too much or too little in your bloodstream. If the day is shortened as it is when you travel east, the dose should be cut. When the trip is westerly and the day is longer, an extra dose of short-acting (when you eat an extra meal) is appropriate. I can't tell you how much to cut or add, that's different for different individuals - ask your doctor.

Worries are very personal and individual things. I'm not a big worrier but I do fret about losing my medications. Solution: I carry two complete sets. One is in that large purse and one is in my suitcase. More insulin, syringes, and swabs are also packed. That way if purse or suitcase are lost or stolen or even forgotten somewhere, I'm not in trouble. There is very little room left in my valise for clothing but then, there are always LAUNDROMATS.

Food is harder to manage. You know how difficult eating in a restaurant can be. Usually you have some understanding of what goes into each dish but what happens when you cross culture lines and you don't know what you're eating? I try to order things without sauces, simply cooked, but it doesn't always work. Then, I figuratively close my eyes and enjoy what is in front of me. Frequent blood sugar finger stick tests and a little more insulin (if needed) get me through.

Oh yes, evening snacks are a problem. Stopping at a restaurant for just a bite is time consuming and annoying. Eateries can't always be found and sometimes they are closed. If the hotel or motel has a coffee shop, I like to stop there. Room service is expensive. I carry cheese and peanut butter cracker packages. They don't need refrigeration or heating and travel quite well. One of those and a glass of water may not be the most enjoyable snack but my needs are filled. Small boxes of raisins also accompany me and allow some flexibility at nosh time. They also, like magnets, bring grandchildren to watch when Grandma unpacks. Their grandma carries such strange things: jelly beans which she won't share, raisins which she will, and that funny kit with the stuff that she pokes her fingers with. I can hear them: "Queer grandma but she's nice."

Now that I've covered your medication and food needs, think about protecting yourself by carrying your doctor's name and phone number, several copies of the medications you take (both generic and proprietary names) and their doses, and a log of your blood sugar values as well as directions for using your blood sugar meter. If you are going abroad information about obtaining emergency medical help and the names and contact data for English-speaking physicians are available from The International Association for Medical Assistance to Travelers, 735 Center St., Lewiston, NY 14092 (phone 716-754-4883).

All packed? Then off you go. Have a wonderful trip.

Diabetic rats or mice don't have to go through all that nonsense. They've been cured. Not us. I often think about changing species but ... remember that when you read about or hear of marvelous new things for diabetics. Usually the research has been done using rodents and we're not rodents. Even if the experimental subjects were humans most of the time there were very few of them. Be patient fellow patients. If the work is valid it will come to your doctor's notice. I review in my mind all the new drugs that have come my way and new procedures as well, to give me faith that this will happen. Reports of islet transplants creep into the papers every once in a while but the techniques are not developed to the point where they can be applied to us. Everybody wishes they were - but they aren't. Just be interested in the news stories but don't get your hopes up. Mice and rats, if they could read, should be more encouraged.

For example, here is a story about preventing IDDM (Type I diabetes) in mice. This form of diabetes develops when the body rejects and destroys part of itself (islet or insulin-producing cells in the pancreas). White blood cells which do the wrecking job are called Tcells. If islet cell antigens (the proteins which T cells identify as part-of-you or not-part-of-you) are put in the thymus (a small gland near the thyroid in the neck) gland when those T cells are maturing, they get identified as part-of-us protein. IDDM is thus, prevented because "self" is recognized as self. I wonder if such a technique would allow the transplantation of foreign islets from the same species or maybe even different species. Lots of islet cells from slaughtered animals are discarded every day. What a waste.

From his desk here in Brooklyn, H. Lebovitz reports on a new medication for Type II (NIDDM - noninsulin dependant diabetics). One group of oral drugs control blood sugar by increasing the amount of insulin produced by the body. These are the sulfonylureas. Biguanidines make insulin work better in the liver and peripheral tissues. The new drug, acarbase, delays the digestion and absorption of carbohydrates.

Carbohydrates. Hmm! In my last column I told you I would learn more about the new approach to diabetic diet and share with you. Counting carbohydrates is the name of the game but the whole approach to them is different. Simple sugars (cakes, cookies, candy, pie) are now believed to be used in the same way as if they were complex carbohydrates (pasta, potatoes, bagels). Go ahead. Enjoy what you once thought of as "a cheat". However, be sure to include it in your count of what you ate. Substitute the new food in your diet plan. Don't just add it. Nobody is telling you that a piece of chocolate cake at every meal is fine but you may have *some* sweets. A new approach to your diet now counts one carbohydrate exchange, one milk exchange, and one fruit exchange as interchangeable. You may have an all fruit meal or a milk meal or any combination you like. The result is a more flexible diet. I am told that control of blood sugar can be managed on the new diet but triglyceride levels may rise. Individualization is the key. Find out what works for *you.*

The American Diabetes Association has published a new set of exchange lists. Look at the new section called "Other Carbohydrate List" and put your tongue back in your mouth. Frosted cake, fruit pie, humus, regular jellies and jams, as well as Danish pastry are allowed. Guilt comes into play here. We've been denied all this good stuff for so long that when it's there in front of you not only will you feel guilty but your loved ones and supporters who challenge you with "You're not allowed that!" must be turned off. Expansion of the Free Food List allows us fat free or reduced fat sour cream, catsup, and fat-free cream cheese to name a few. These are major changes in diabetic menus and I urge you to buy a copy of the new publication. I will also urge you to enjoy your new found freedom.

Rats and mice have not achieved what we have achieved. They are still limited to those dull-looking pellets. I guess I'm glad to still remain in my species.

Medical ethics became an active discipline once the original "Who Shall Live?" decisions in the pioneer Seattle program had to be faced in the early years of dialysis therapy. In the present era with funding for all who desire treatment, derivative ethical questions have arisen. In 1994, as one of several respondents to a series of difficult questions prepared for a textbook on medical ethics, Barry submitted the following answers.

Medical Ethics

A patient threatens legal action if not permitted to withdraw from dialytic therapy

When the threat of legal action is more important than granting the wish of a patient, there is something wrong with our priorities. Unfortunately, the desire to allow life to end, is thought to be a result of mental incompetence. A decision to continue life, no matter how painful, embarrassing, or without pleasure that life is, is accepted as coming from a healthy mind. If the decision is to allow natural events to end life, mental ability and stability are questioned. Ceasing dialysis is not *pure suicide*. It is rather, recognition of the inevitable end to life. Dialysis is not without pain, discomfort, and the expenditure of much energy. Consider only the effort of an outpatient to arrive at a dialysis unit.

Pushed by circumstances, what many people dread is an aware mind trapped in an incompetent body. Some may regard their "quality of life" as negative. Life belongs to the individual and just as we accept the individual's right to make many decisions (marriage, bearing children), so must we accept the right to decide to refuse therapy. We each are in charge of one life, our own. Recognition of this is inherent in the endorsement of Living Wills.

Should dialysis be continued for a combative mentally defective patient?

Treatment is meant to help patients, to improve quality of life. The Hippocratic Oath states that physicians should do no harm. In every case, a balance between improving an existing medical condition and causing distress, possibly pain, and fear - must be struck. The patient is obviously troubled - she struggles. She is being harmed. Even if there is a functioning mind deep within, comprehension cannot be there. A reasonable assumption is that no one has explained what is happening to her.

When therapy may cure a medical problem, a reason to continue treatment might exist. In the absence of such hope, dialysis only prolongs and deepens the misery of the patient. Discontinuing dialysis when there is no future would not be euthanasia but only recognizing that death is the result of kidney failure. Cost of maintaining life should also be considered. The nation can no longer provide *all available* medical treatment to everyone. Decisions regarding who to treat and who not to treat, must be made. Money should be spent with common sense.

Let me say here that if sufficient funds to treat all the ill were available, I would still agree with a responsible nephrologist's decision to no longer dialyze a hopelessly impaired intellectually vegetative patient. My primary grounds are compassion and a desire to improve the quality of life. Strange, but at times quality of life is bettered by death.

Must dialysis be continued for a disruptive combative woman?

Responsibility lies across the shoulders of health care providers and also across the shoulders of patients. People who distract those taking care of them, interfere with more than comfort of others in a dialysis unit. People who are distracted and stressed do not function as well as they should. Squeaky wheels get the grease and so the disruptive get the attention. Each of us has only so much time and energy to spend on our jobs. Therefore, care for the compliant, cooperative patient is downgraded. "Good" patients are essentially punished to benefit "bad" ones.

Certainly attempts to treat disruptive patients should be made but these people cannot be allowed to constantly discomfort others around them. I would begin by documenting her behavior. Tapes, films, videos of her actions would constitute legal proof of her conduct. The next step might be an attempt to isolate her in the dialysis clinic. If this did not work, she should certainly be transferred to another facility using the procedure detailed.

Staff could explain to her (probably unsuccessfully), that while she feels comfortable, others do not. The reaction she is faced with is a consequence of her actions. She has not lived up to her responsibilities as a patient. Patient responsibility should be clearly explained.

Other alternatives should be explored. Independent wealth might allow her to design a comfortable, friendly environment in her home. A sympathetic person sharing a good relationship with the patient, might be able to engross her in designing a home unit. Involvement in her own care could potentially change her behavior.

In summary, explanations, isolation, and involvement should be attempted. If success does not come to pass then I would agree to legally discharging her with notice. No one patient is more important than others.

A vascular surgeon refuses to repair the vascular access of a drug addict who repeatedly destroys his dialysis access by self-injection of heroin?

Young men such as this, long ago declared themselves to be beyond redemption. While his background is not detailed, surely reasons for his behavior can be found. However, many other people have overcome similar circumstances and become valued members of society. If questioned, he would know that his behavior was wrong. His choice was to continue this kind of activity. His choice now is to commit slow suicide. Many chances to conform to normal rules of living have been afforded him. I cite the attempts to reach him, provide dialysis treatment, and the creation of three access sites.

Surgeons seldom sit around. There is plenty for them to do and asking them to use valuable time, OR space, and material on what will undoubtedly be thwarted efforts is senseless.

Rehabilitation treatment should be offered to the patient. If he displays any attempt to learn positive behavior, he should be encouraged and even given another access. If he does not, there is no hope for him. Proof of his ability to be concerned for himself and take helpful action is inherent in his arriving at a dialysis unit.

We spend much time, money, and energy on people who give nothing to our world. They are not worthless but so many others are worth more. Let us put increased exertions into public education, care for old people, feeding the hungry,...

The responsible vascular surgeon is correct in refusing further vascular surgery and is compassionate in basing *his* decision on the patient's decision.

Should dialysis be started for a patient dying from AIDS whose life is not salvageable?

No hope exists that dialysis would save the life of a man with a disease that leads in 99.9% of its victims, to death. His wishes are not delineated in this presentation.

Honoring the desires of a patient does not exist as the single deciding factor when a diagnosis of AIDS exists. Other people, patients and health care providers, would be involved if he was dialyzed. A potential for mistakes exists. If I was a dialysis patient, I would refuse to be dialyzed on a machine previously used for an AIDS patient. My right is to know if that artificial kidney had been so used. Isolating certain equipment for use only with AIDS patients would eliminate the problem. Such isolation, however, would not remove danger to the health care professionals who come in contact with fluids from the patient. Risk of infection is present. Stress on the workers is increased. Concern for patients is important but so is concern for those who take care of them.

Application of medical techniques to those who should not be treated is an ethical issue troubling many. Each must make his own decision and mine is to not treat people who are beyond help. Once begun on therapy it is difficult to discontinue. More humane is the judgment to not begin. The nephrologist is correct.

After a stroke, heart attack, and respiratory failure requiring placement of an endotracheal tube for respiration in an 82 year old man should dialysis be begun?

In a case like this, I argue with the concept of *necessitated placement of an endotracheal tube.* Two systems had failed - coronary arteries and brain circulation. Seventy-two years is not a short life. The body was deteriorating. Death is the natural end of life and should be allowed to occur when it comes, without interference.

Another system failed and again invasive therapy was performed. That was wrong. Iatrogenic kidney failure then occurred and was presented to the nephrologist for treatment. The patient should not have been pushed so far down the road. If her life had not been mechanically prolonged, the nephrologist would not have been faced with the decision to treat or not treat her.

The nephrologist who decides negatively makes a wise judgement to no longer lengthen what had become an existence not a life.

A medical chief fires a woman resident who refuses to care for HIV+ patients in fear for her children

Conscientious objectors were allowed to not participate in battle situations but to serve their country in other ways. Physician refusal to treat HIV+ patients may be considered in the same light.

The question is whether people who have taken an oath to serve others may pick and choose who they will serve.

Perhaps doctors with strong convictions that they should not be forced to treat HIV+ patients should leave the profession and find new careers. Perhaps they should change to a specialty where less threat exists. Ophthalmology and psychiatry come to mind.

What is not arguable is her right to morally judge her patients and decide which ones to treat. Fear of HIV is understandable. A woman in the midst of her child bearing years may well be more concerned than a male of the same age. Consideration of an unborn does not seem to have been raised by the resident but it is in my mind. My belief in the right of each of us to control our own lives comes into play here. Along with that right is the necessity to live with the results of our decisions.

The Chief of the Medical Service is correct in his decision. No compromise seems possible. Medical residents can give no less than full care to the people in their charge and at this stage in their training they cannot decide who will and who will not be under their care.

An anesthesiologist refuses his service for an unrelated friend of a kidney patient who volunteers to give his kidney

If the anesthesiologist would also refuse to involve himself in a living *related* organ donor transplant, logic would be on his side. If he would not, his bias is showing.

Living organ donors are at minimal risk. Adverse effects are seldom noted. The possibility of maintaining healthy life with much less renal capacity than that provided by a pair of normally functioning kidneys is beyond dispute. Physiologically no reason exists to deny a friend the chance to rehabilitate a loved one.

Our society allows blood donation, egg donation, and sperm donation from living volunteers. Kidney donation is an extension of such actions. Because no payment is involved, the offered organ is a gift, not a sale, and is altruistically motivated. We do not question the propriety of allowing parts of the dead to continue life. Why question ongoing life for two people?

The anesthesiologist is wrong and should be encouraged to rethink his decision. If he still retains his opinion then, perhaps, he should remove himself from working on any transplant case.

An Arab prince offers a new hospital wing for rapid receipt of a cadaver kidney out of turn

I would hope that the hospital involved turned down the suggestion of trading a cadaver kidney for a hospital wing in favor of other proposals. In some nations kidneys can be bought. Whether or not you agree with the morality of the sale, it exists, and the Arabian prince can take advantage of it. If he further insists on American know-how and skills to perform the operation, he may try to make arrangements for the physicians of his choice to be temporarily licensed in the foreign nation. It would probably not be allowed.

The patient and her husband are then left with the prospect of continued hemodialysis. Good years on dialysis are possible and using his money wisely, the prince should arrange construction of a pleasant, even elegant, dialysis arrangement in their home. Furthermore, financing excellent training for several dialysis technicians would insure excellent medical care. Introducing the couple to patients who have lived on dialysis for many years and who maintain good quality of life, might teach them the possibility of such a course.

Money entitles people to the best available care. It does not make them more worthwhile than others. The hospital should not allow itself to be bought.

A teen age child volunteers her kidney for her depressed diabetic father

People who will eventually become diabetic should not consider donating a kidney and certainly should not be coerced to do so. The father's lack of concern for his daughter, his self-concern, his belief that his life is somehow more important than hers, should be discussed with parent and child. Also noted is his status as a noncompliant patient. Failure to follow rules will jeopardize any new kidney he receives.

While it is depressing to go through the hard times of poor response to treatment and a long wait for an organ, many other patients have survived similar circumstances. Treat the depression. Stress the value of compliance. Gently point out that he is the architect of many of his problems. Teach him the realities of diabetes.

Another factor to consider is that his daughter is in her child bearing years. In a diabetic family, the next generation will probably be diabetic as well. If our prediabetic Type II has children who are Type I (as happens) those children might have diabetic kidney failure earlier in their lives. If mother insists on being a kidney donor, she probably would choose to give to her offspring rather than to the man she sprang from.

The dilemma is partly moral and partly medical. On both counts I vote against the procedure and agree with the endocrinologist.

A New York merchant on dialysis requests referral to India to purchase a kidney

Kidney purchase is marginally illegal in India and so the patient is breaking no law in opting for this course. Nothing is kept secret. He has a right to a copy of his medical history and the Indian physicians may read it and summarize.

As to resuming care of a patient after treatment in another facility, if the transplant was performed in a United States hospital, collaboration would be forthcoming.

Patient benefit, patient healing, are the aim of the doctor. Adjusting medications or procedures provided by a second physician is acceptable. Therefore, resuming care of a patient is permissible.

Preserving your own life, seeking any kind of legal treatment, is the patient's right. The nephrologist should be complimented that the man is satisfied with her care and again wishes to place his life in her hands. She is wrong in judging her patient's decision and refusing him treatment.

A kidney from a mentally defective and noncomprehending sibling is to be transplanted

A few years ago a child was conceived for the stated purpose of becoming a bone marrow donor for an older sister. When the new daughter was old enough she indeed gave bone marrow and saved her sister's life. This case proposes using a mentally deficient sibling as a kidney donor. Both dilemmas raise the same question.

Parents are legally responsible for decisions affecting both proposed donors. Arguing that their conclusions are those that would be made by the immature sisters if they were mentally responsible, seems illogical. There is no way of knowing what the girls would decide if they were adult. Accountability for the conclusions rests on the parents.

Kidney donation and bone marrow donation are minimally physically risky for the donors. Psychological gains may lie in the future for both girls. Gratitude from the recipients may foster closer relationships. More attention may be paid to the givers. In a family where one child is sick and the other well, the sick one receives more attention. When the differences between siblings are made more equal, concern for them will even out.

Under these circumstances the moral question lies before the ill daughters. When they ask for the donation they signal their resolution of the problem. A feeling of guilt will probably remain for the rest of their lives. Guilt is not always avoidable or bad. Out in the open and discussed, it can be dealt with.

My moral judgement would be different but I do not disagree with the decision.

Should the President or the Pope be given priority in receiving a cadaver organ?

Organs are normally allocated on a point system which takes into account age and prognosis among other things. There is no reason for any man to be treated differently from other potential recipients. If the usual procedure was followed, arguments about favoritism would be negated.

Even for the president no valid reason for placing him first on the list would exist. Indeed, a sick president, recovering from major surgery, might well be expected to resign. Similarly, an ill state governor should keep the well-being of his state in mind and leave his post with or without surgery.

Some of Barry's best writing were her last columns including this 1997 excerpt from Diabetic Directions in which she tries to make sense out of disparate reports.

Diabetic Directions: Type

The diagnosis has been made. DIABETES. You feel a little more self-assured. It's almost always better to have an answer than to be up in the air. You start paying attention to the words people say. "My aunt had a little touch of sugar." "Maybe you have the gentler kind of diabetes." "I hope you won't have to take shotsl"

Further lab test results come back. Your doctor tells you that the type of diabetes you have is not clear. You sit up. What is going on here?

Well, to start with there is no such thing as a little touch of sugar. That's like being a little bit pregnant.

Diabetes can bc defined as an inability of the body to metabolize (burn) glucose (sugar) normally. Glucose is important because it is the fuel or source of energy, that runs all the body's activities. Reasons for this abnormality vary. Understand the mechanisms.

No matter what kind of diabetes you have, insulin is the important hormone. Made by the beta cells in the islets of Langerhans in the pancreas, insulin's job is to get glucose into body cells. Not all the body cells need insulin to accomplish this. Cells in the glomeruli of the kidney, the retina of the eye and nerve cells allow sugar to enter with no help from insulin. For this reason the level of sugar in these cells is equal to the level of sugar in the plasma. When blood sugar is high, sugar inside these cells is equally high and it is now believed that elevated glucose levels cause diabetic complications. Other body cells do without sugar when insulin is not present or can't work. Absence of insulin is due to the destruction of the pancreatic beta cells or loss of the whole organ caused by disease or surgery. The body rejects and destroys its own cells in an autoimmune process. When enough cells have been blown away, diabetes is the result. This is called Type 1 or Juvenile Diabetes or IDDM (Insulin Dependant Diabetes Mellitus). Type 2 or Maturity Onset Diabetes of NIDDM (Noninsulin Dependent Diabetes Mellitus) occurs when insulin doesn't work right. All the cells except retina, glomerular, and nerve cells have receptors on their surfaces. I call these "grabbers". Grabbers grab insulin from the plasma and, next, the insulin grabs sugar from the plasma. All of this then turns around and pokes the sugar into the cell where it is burned to fuel everything the body does.

A recent paper by Takeshi Kuzuya, MD of Japan is very exciting because it puts all the kinds of diabetes in a logical order. He states that Type 1 diabetes is the only variety in its category. Defined as insulin requiring diabetes (no substitutions - you die without it), Type 1 stands alone.

A major confusion exists defining *insulin-requiring and insulin-taking* diabetics. The first is Type 1 and the second is Type 2 treated with insulin. Diet, exercise, weight loss, oral medications may control sugar in these cases without insulin. Now let's go on.

The other kinds are all Type 2. Gestational, MODY, insulin-taking, J diabetes, Flatbush diabetes, impaired glucose tolerance, and steroid diabetes as well as the Type 2 that is common in Japan. You may never have heard of these illnesses so let me make a simple list.
Gestational diabetes begins in the second trimester of pregnancy because of a growth spurt of the fetus that requires the mother to produce more insulin. She cannot, so there is a shortage of insulin. It usually disappears with the birth of the child but may return as Type 2 in later years.

MODY explains itself when we clarify the initials as Maturity Onset Diabetes of the Young. Teens and preteens who fit the profile for Type 2 make up this group.
Insulin-taking Diabetics are Type 2s whose blood glucose is not controlled with oral agents.

J Diabetes is named for Jamaica. Teenagers in this heritage group may present as type 1s but they later fit the Type 2 criteria.
Flatbush Diabetics are Type 2s with ketoacidosis (high sugar levels cause ketone bodies to appear in the blood of many Type 1s).
Steroid Diabetes is caused by the administration of steroids and disappears when they are no longer taken.
Japanese Type 2s are thin people.
Impaired Glucose Tolerance is not defined as diabetes but may be a precursor.
Latent Autoimmune Diabetes in Adults is due to slowly progressive destruction of beta cells that can stop before it is complete.

Exceptions to explanations exist. I am an example. My Gestational diabetes went on to become Type 1 not Type 2.

In order to classify diabetes the following must be considered. Age of onset, fast or slow onset, obesity, ketones, stability of blood glucose, family history, specific HLA or tissue types, islet cell and insulin and anti-GAD antibodies, other autoimmune diseases, C-peptide levels, and a need for insulin treatment are all important.

A little touch of diabetes? You bet. Accurate diagnosis and treatment to enable control of blood sugar and blood pressure is what it's all about. Uncontrolled diabetes can lead to severe complications including heart attacks and strokes. Loss of vision, loss of kidney function, and all the manifestations of neuropathy interfere with quality of life. Diabetes seems to affect every cell, every function of the body. Don't give up hope. Research sheds light on understanding and coping and living in a chronic disease state.

****

Two new developments leap out at me. In Denver, D.R. Fleming's group showed that injecting insulin *through* clothing was fine. No infections resulted. They went through material as thick as denim. More frequent bruising and bloodstains on clothing occurred. When eating in restaurants, less attention from strangers is a side effect. This allows me to take my shots in my abdomen, which I prefer, to using my arms or thighs. Life is a little more pleasant.

A new fast-acting insulin is on the market. Named “lispro” it reduces the rise in blood sugar after eating and lowers the number of hypoglycemic episodes. Too many insulin reactions seem to destroy awareness of low blood sugar and that can be dangerous. Reducing the quantity of such episodes returns perception of low or lowering glucose. A danger not considered by the manufacturer, is the addition of a new kind of insulin to the already existing insulins. Insulin vials are not marked so they can be told apart by feel and the blind or visually impaired diabetic may unwittingly use the wrong kind. Several years have gone by and we cannot convince the insulin producers to mark the bottles. Any suggestions for how to get them to cooperate?

Speaking of lowering the number of insulin reactions, pancreas transplants certainly do that. The body responds to low blood sugar by excreting epinephrine. Patients with pancreas grafts show a release of epinephrine but not the same quantity as a normal response. Symptoms of low blood sugar are based on autonomic neuropathy.

Successful transplants are great but there is still much we don’t understand. Cultured testicular cells and purified islet cells transplanted under the kidney capsule showed prolonged graft survival without immunosuppression. Implanting foreign cells into the testes is also a safe place for them. What is special about the testes? There may be something special about the reproductive tract. After all, women don’t reject the babies in their wombs and that is surely a foreign body.

However, this kind of thinking may be due to a low blood sugar on my part. Why? Blood flow to the brain does not increase until the sugar level is very low and that alters cognitive function. I knew there had to be an explanation for my occasional crazinesses.

Barry in this 1995 column weighs the unique concerns of facing holidays when abundant food and relaxation are the rule for others but denied to those with diabetes. She proposes: "Think about your behavior. ...Does your conversation always lean on what is wrong with you? Try answering "I'm just fine." when they ask how you are and ask how the important things in their lives are. Find something you can do to help. Even people confined to wheelchairs can fold napkins or, sitting at a table, clean vegetables. Plan far ahead and learn one good joke to tell. If you want to be warmly welcomed, don't criticize. ... Support the people around you, they will like you better. If that's too hard, put a smile on your face and sit there quietly. If you can't do that, leave the room for a while. ... A hug, a kiss, and a warm "Thank you for a lovely time." combine to construct a good aura and possibly a return invitation."

HOLIDAYS

It's not news to you that holidays are depressing times for many people. Loneliness and missing loved ones contribute. If a longed for contact is not made, we can feel ignored, unwanted. If you are depressed you probably won't reach out and must be approached by others. Other problems can also cause trouble. Us diabetics may be just plain hungry.

Heaps and heaps of food, some of which doesn't fit into diabetic diets, served at times that are not on our usual eating schedule - in simple words: heaps and heaps of problems. No matter which strategy you pick to deal with holiday food, you will probably be left with a sense of annoyance if not guilt.

Living with the need to control yourself every time you open your mouth to eat, is not natural and doesn't come easy. Everyone has periods when they are not hungry and intervals when they think starvation is around the corner. As diabetics we are expected to treat both conditions the same and eat the same amount of food in the same proportions of protein, carbohydrates, dairy products, and fruits and vegetables as well as fats. Not only are we asked to regulate that kind of stuff, but we are required to consume these foods at regulated hours of the day. No way, Jose.

Now hold on a minute. Here I am whining and complaining and that's not the way to give a situation a positive twist and make holidays happy. Something must be changed. Let's redo the surroundings. Find a way around the food problem.

If a diet is prescribed that demands a way of life that doesn't satisfy or make happy the person it is set out for, you may expect noncompliance. So when it comes to holidays, there has to be a way that is acceptable. I guess I have chosen as my way of dealing with nutrition stresses, educated cheating. Playing around with the rules means that you have to understand the regulations.

Basically I want to keep my blood sugar under reasonable control, because if I don't, I won't feel good. Losing control of blood glucose for a short time will not kill me but it may make me uncomfortable.

I'll start discussing what I find most difficult to deal with and that is poor timing of meals. Anger is always my reaction to an invitation for brunch, or for a large repast in the middle of the afternoon or a late night supper. Those don't fit my eating schedule. The rest of the world is not on my consumption timetable and it is not fair for me to ask them to do things my way. So I complain to myself, grumble a little, and with a smile, accept the invitation and say "I'd love to come." My shifted dining plans require extra insulin injections because my intermediate acting insulin must be taken at the usual times so the doses overlap as they should. The fast acting insulin will be injected 30 minutes before I expect to eat. If brunch is scheduled early, I count it as breakfast. If it is close to lunch, OK I treat it like lunch and have had breakfast. Midafternoon feasts require more insulin and less food than is offered. Hostesses frequently don't understand, but that's the way it is. Of course when I get home, I eat supper and I really don't feel like it. Late night banquets have me combining supper calories with late night snack calories and that can be good especially if I'm enjoying the feast. Sometimes I'm even lucky and the meal is served at a time that is good for me. Frequently this happens when I am the cook.

Your major problem may be facing a table stacked high with things you love to eat but shouldn't. Study the display. Let your taste buds do the walking. Figure out which of the forbidden items is the most favorite. (Maybe even choose two.) Keep your serving sizes in mind. Be good. But, and that's a big BUT, indulge. Enjoy. Don't feel guilty. And don't repeat the cheat at every meal or even every day. Pat your tummy. Keep the taste in your mouth. Smile.

I say I'm glad to be diabetic today not twenty years ago. Sugar substitutes, diet drinks, and other low sugar offerings (I will take a break in five minutes and go indulge in a sugar free Popsicle) make life more pleasant than it used to be. Grin. The ADA has just made it more agreeable once again. Carbohydrate intake is liberalized. A recommendation is on board that we count the number of carbohydrate exchanges we consume and use that figure to control our food intake. Moreover, they say that we can count simple sugars (yup - sugar) and complex carbohydrates (pasta, potato, cereal) as equals. Nobody is saying have a large slice of chocolate cake whenever you want to or don't count it in your diet prescription, but there is a liberalization of what diabetics can eat. I have already told you more than I know on this subject but will keep reading and listening and will write more when I know more. Meanwhile, just ease up a little.

Food dilemmas are not the only depressing things that occur during holidays. How can you make these special days happier for yourself? Give out a lot of hugs and kisses. Save some for yourself. Balance what you should do with pleasure activities. Don't feel sorry for yourself. You are still here. Don't make others uncomfortable by discussing personal problems too long. Everybody has personal problems.

I've been talking about food but then I'm a diabetic and food is very important in my life. Holidays, however, include many other things. Try to spend them with people you like but if that isn't possible be with somebody that you at least should like: yourself. Get out of the house. Go to a movie, a concert, a play. Plan to sit or walk someplace you like that is safe (I live in a big city) for you when you are alone. Try the zoo or a museum.

Share with others. Have you ever volunteered? It's a rewarding activity. Think how good you could feel rocking a child who lives in an institution. They hug back almost immediately. Read a little one a book that you brought and then give it as a keepsake. Play tic-tac-toe with a kid - over and over and over again. I'll bet they still want more. Make it fun. Instead of x's and o's, play with belly buttons and toes. Find out what kind of treat they can have with their next meal and provide it. An orange may not seem like much to you but it sure can be.

Volunteer for a helpful hot line. Just being ears for a troubled person is a good thing to do and you may learn that there are others worse off than you.

Old age homes can provide the same sense of awareness for where you are in life. Play cards, read a story, help feed, give a shampoo, scratch an itching back, sing a song, take a walk, push a wheelchair. There are a million things to do if you let your mind go. Manicures are good for both men and women (no, don't put purple polish on him unless he really wants it). Bring glue and paper plates and make silly hats. Maybe you can even stay for supper. Then look around. The holiday is finished and you made it good not only for yourself but for others. That's great. Now start thinking about the next one coming up.

It's possible that I've gone too far and that you are going to spend time with people you love. Think about your behavior. Are you a person others get concerned about. Does your conversation always lean on what is wrong with you? Try answering "I'm just fine" when they ask how you are and ask how the important things in their lives are. Find something you can do to help. Even people confined to wheelchairs can fold napkins or, sitting at a table, clean vegetables.

Plan far ahead and learn one good joke to tell. If you want to be warmly welcomed, don't criticize. I can think of *no* situations which can be handled in only one correct way. Support the people around you, they will like you better. If that's too hard, put a smile on your face and sit there quietly. If you can't do that, leave the room for a while. The object is to make yourself liked better and the only guy you have control of, is, you guessed it, number one. A hug, a kiss, and a warm "Thank you for a lovely time." combine to construct a good aura and possibly a return invitation.

Holidays. Some are easier to cope with. Few people are saddened by Flag Day. Thanksgiving is harder. Depression makes difficult times harder still but remember depression can be part of a healing process. There are good, legitimate reasons for being in the middle of a slump. It may be best to accept where you are - this time.

Readers of Barry's column in 1991 were briefed on the introduction of tacrolimus (FK-506) and erythropoietin, as well as the potential value of blocking advanced glycosylated end-products (AGEs) with aminoguanidine as a means of preventing diabetic complications. Presenting these complex subjects to a lay audience was precisely the challenge that Barry met so well.

ALWAYS SOMETHING NEW

Humans, it seems to me, are always looking for something new to cure or at least improve, their aches and pains. All over the world, people have tried, and use, animal and plant tissues or products to accomplish health goals. Present day lists contain many, many drugs some of which are man made and some of which are not. Because scientists can define the exact chemical composition of most of these substances, what their origins are no longer matters, but still there is an interest.

The story goes that the Sandoz Corporation - a huge Swiss pharmaceutical company, suggested that workers bring back samples of soil from strange places they found themselves in - probably on vacation. And so, a fungus, with interesting properties, was discovered in a little bit of earth taken from a plateau above a fjord in Norway. A product of that fungus is known to you as cyclosporine. Transplant recipients are glad for this piece of history as are people with certain other medical problems (cyclosporine fights things besides rejection such as a parasite infection known as Schistosomiasis). Cyclosporine, when first used, was hailed as the great solution to problems of rejection, but as time passed, side effects, some of which are bad, were seen. A miracle cure had not been found. The search went on.

Another fungus with an antirejection product came to the attention of doctors, this time in Japan. Again there was hopeful speculation that the new medication would be the best of all possible immunosuppressive agents. FK 506 works well. Rejections, not reversed by other methods, are often resolved with FK 506, particularly in liver transplantation, where 7 of 10 patients, as reported by Starzl and his group, in the journal *the Lancet* in 1989, had successful outcomes. Other antirejection regimens had been tried. An advantage with FK 506 treatment is the possible dose lowering or even elimination of steroid therapy.

Unfortunately, like cyclosporine, FK 506 can damage kidneys and nerves, and can cause diabetes, but these side effects are not as strong with FK 506 as with cyclosporine. Cholesterol levels lower and blood pressure doesn't rise during FK 506 treatment. Growth of hair and overgrowth of gums are absent. FK 506 administration has been quite effective in liver, heart, lung, and combinations of these, grafts. The best doses of the drug have been established for transplants of these organs. Kidney grafting with FK 506 is also effective but the selection of amounts of medication have yet to be established. In part, the failure to determine preferred drug levels is due to the kind of patients first chosen.

Generally, when human experimentation is done the most desperately ill patients are dealt with first causing less than optimal results. Time passes and sufferers in better condition are administered the investigative drugs. Results improve if the drug is a good one. Following this logic, the 36 kidney graft recipients chosen by Starzl et al. to receive FK 506 were all difficult to graft. Many of them were highly sensitized to multiple tissue antigens, 10 were undergoing kidney retransplantation, 10 also underwent liver transplantation at an earlier time (6 patients) or concomitantly (4 patients), and 2 patients received a third organ (heart or pancreas) in addition to a liver and kidney. After 4 to 13 months all but 2 of the 36 were alive, 29 were dialysis free and most had good renal function. Of the 29 dialysis free patients, 20 took little or no steroid. Cellular rejection was responsible for the loss of one kidney and irreversible humoral rejection was present in 3 of the 9 who had had antidonor cytotoxic antibodies.

The next step in evaluating FK 506 is to determine the optimal doses for kidney transplantation. There will be changes in how today's immunosuppressive drugs (imuran, cyclosporine, FK 506, prednisone) are used. Their combinations, timing, and doses will vary but the greatest modifications will come each time a new medication appears on the scene.

Care and cure of diabetes comprises another health setting where an active search for new treatments is underway. Before one can say maybe this new substance will help, understanding of the process one wishes to interfere with is necessary.

Glycosylation is the hottest new theory explaining why high blood sugar causes diabetic complications. It is a two part chemical reaction. At first, glucose and protein combine, without the aid of enzymes, to form glycosylated protein. The more glucose present, the more glycosylated protein is formed. Next, these rather big molecules join together to form large clumps or aggregates of sticky matter. Such joining is irreversible and occurs in the blood stream and tissues. Advanced glycosylation end products (AGEs) is the name given to the aggregates. AGEs are believed to cause many problems. For instance, AGEs on the walls of blood vessels keep nitric oxide, produced by the body, from relaxing and widening blood vessels, thus playing a role in the production of high blood pressure. Fluid flowing through rigid pipes exerts greater pressure than that moving through elastic ones. Cross-linking of arterial wall connective tissue protein has been shown. Stiffness also plays a part in diabetic circulation. Erythrocyte (red blood cell) membranes become glycosylated and as a consequence the cells grow more rigid. Stiffness of circulating cells contributes to circulatory problems. Capillaries (the smallest blood vessels) are quite tiny and the red blood cells are slightly larger in diameter. Therefore, in order to get through the capillaries the cells must flex and squeeze. When they cannot do that, the circulatory system is blocked. Not a good situation. Another membrane which is glycated is that known as the glomerular basement membrane located in the kidney. Alterations in the glomerular basement membrane when its proteins are glycated include changes in physicochemical and binding properties (other substances bind to the structure in order that they may work). One of the substances present in glomerular basement membranes is collagen. Whether or not modifications such as glycosylation of kidney cell membranes bring about diabetic kidney disease is not yet clear.

As an aside, collagen becomes glycosylated and cross links forming browning products. These compounds develop in everyone, accumulate with aging, and in diabetes although a connection between their buildup and the occurrence of diabetic complications has not been made. Still, notice must be taken that diabetic bodies often seem to be aged beyond their years.

In rats, cataracts due to aging (senile cataracts) and due to diabetes both show increased amounts of glycated (glycosylated) crystallin.

Macrophages (white blood cells) have receptor sites which bind to glycosylated proteins and aid in their ingestion removing them from the body but large amounts of AGEs may saturate these receptors and accumulate.

The major biological effects of excessive nonenzymatic glycosylation include: inactivation of enzymes; inhibition of regulatory molecule binding; crosslinking of glycosylated proteins and trapping of soluble proteins by glycosylated extracellular matrix (both may progress in the absence of glucose); decreased susceptibility to proteolysis (breakdown of proteins); abnormalities of nucleic acid function (glucose also attaches to nucleic acids); altered macromolecular recognition and phagocytosis; and increased ability to cause an immune response.

Names to remember as contributors to our understanding of AGE are Brownlee, Vlassara, and Cerami. Among other things they have shown the susceptibility of fibrin to degradation by the specific fibrinolytic (destroys fibrin) enzyme plasmin. Plasmin decreases fibrin. This also occurs when a specific amino acid in plasmin (lysine) is chemically altered by the processes called acetylation or carbamylation as well as glycosylation. Decreased degradation of fibrin may contribute to the accumulation of fibrin and several other proteins observed in those tissues most frequently affected by the complications of diabetes.

All the quoted observations point to the likelihood that clumping of cross linked glycosylated proteins may be one cause of diabetic complications. If the development of AGE clumps can be stopped there is hope that newly diagnosed diabetics may avoid eye, kidney, nerve, arteriovascular and heart problems. Aminoguanidine is a drug that stops the cross linking in diabetic rats and dogs. Even now investigations in humans are progressing. It is too early to come to conclusions but hope is high.

Glycosylated hemoglobin is used to measure the quantity of glucose over the previous 2 months in the blood of diabetics. Red blood cells contain hemoglobin and their life span is approximately 2 months. Glycosylated hemoglobin can't un-glycosylate so the amount present reflects the total of sugar in the blood stream for that length of time. If the glycosylated hemoglobin measured is the simple, unlinked form, the administration of aminoguanidine will not interfere with this measure of glycemic control. However, if what is measured is the crosslinked variety, aminoguanidine will prevent this assay from being a logical means of learning about patient's diabetic control. Another way will need to be found. Seeking something new will keep lab people busy.

Finding new things shifts situations around. Well, erythropoietin really wasn't new but the method of producing it was. Erythropoietin as a kidney produced hormone which stimulates bone marrow to produce red blood cells has been known about for years and the possibility of curing anemia with erythropoietin is not a new thought. Obtaining large enough quantities to make treatment feasible has been the difficulty. Erythropoietin is produced naturally in very small amounts. With the advent of genetic engineering, bacteria can be forced to produce EPO (as it is fondly known) by the bathtub.

Dialysis patients who previously needed frequent blood transfusions, now receive EPO and are freed from a procedure which leaves them open to the hazard of contracting hepatitis and AIDS from contaminated blood. Unlike FK 506, the negative side effects of EPO are few. Positive side effects are intricately mixed with those produced by the alleviation of anemia. They include an increase in the sense of well being (84%), better appetite (81%), improvement in sexual function (62%), socializing (70%), sleep (68%), skin color (51%), and increased exercise capacity (78%). Improved mental functioning is reported. The author must report her observation of a strange bad side effect - broken bones due to such an exuberance of good feeling on the part of EPO treated patients that they ran and fell or tripped and went down.

As you may know, a certain percentage of people with successful renal grafts exhibit high hematocrits. Erythropoietin production by their diseased kidneys added to that from their new kidney has been thought of as an explanation but if that is so, dialysis patients who retain their failed kidneys should not need transfusions and that is not true. The picture appears to be complicated with other factors involved. Just one of my thoughts.

Two negative side effects have been reported with EPO therapy - hypertension (which can be controlled) and in a small number of patients, convulsions (which have resulted in no harm). A careful comparison of renal failure patients treated with and without EPO showed no difference in the number of convulsions. Anemic peritoneal dialysis patients seem to benefit as well as anemic hemodialysis patients. An added benefit occurs when pretreatment anemic uremic people are given erythropoietin - they do not become sensitized to other human antigens as they do when transfused and so are easier to match with cadaveric organs.

EPO stands as an uncomplicated drug to administer. Given either as an intravenous or a subcutaneous injection, hematocrit levels respond within 4 to 12 weeks by increasing in direct relationship to the size of the dose. Higher levels of hemoglobin can be achieved gradually allowing the body time to adjust. EPO represents a striking and wonderful advance in the search for new cures.

There are many diseases and many difficulties in renal failure and diabetes which still need new approaches and new drugs. Thank heavens the urge to find novel treatments continues. What will the future hold?

Admitting that "Living with diabetes, as living with any chronic disease, is hard," Barry, in 1991, dissects the impact of depression on the diabetic individual and his or her spouse and family. While small children subjected to fingerstick blood testing escape depression because they know no other life style, their parents react to the gravity of a lifelong affliction with gloom. Recognizing the inevitability of depression, Barry advises striving "to make it short. Perhaps it serves a purpose." Characteristic of her style, Barry cited key sources.

Depressing Diabetes

When I decided to write about diabetes and depression I mulled it over for a while and it seemed to me that certain things were self-evident. Of course, when you have diabetes you get depressed. Nobody wants to be sick. There is an exception to illness-awareness depression - the small child who doesn't know that all small children don't get their fingers stuck for blood, don't get injections before they eat, and can eat whatever they want, whenever they want. These children don't get depressed over their condition. Knowledge of normalcy comes soon enough.

Depression over a changed life style, over a deteriorating body, must be almost a standard thing. When complications set in, blue moods probably deepen. Loss of vision (total or less), kidney failure, amputation of a leg or finger, altered sex life, inability to work, pain that won't go away, that there is nothing to do for, uncontrollable blood sugar - all are good and legitimate reasons for depression. Realizing that you are trapped within a failing body is no cause for rejoicing.

And then there are those around you. Parents living with a diabetic child have down times. A spouse or significant other can be less than happy with their changed living conditions or for their ill one. Who does it affect when the mother in a family is sick? How about friends? How do they react? Mine are wonderful - asking me what time I'd like to eat and going along, pleasantly, with my requests. But some friends cannot deal with illness and break the relationship, undoubtedly causing depression in both people.

Depression comes from strange things, too. My syringes are ordered by the thousand and when that box is delivered and I know that each of those needles will pierce my skin three times for a total of three thousand sticks - I do get blue.

The rest of life, that not dealing with diabetes, is rich with disappointments and bad happenings. More reasons for depression.

Approximately 2 out of 10 diabetics have been found to be depressed at any one time but I think those numbers should be looked at in a different way. Depression comes and goes, it may be present one moment and absent the next. We can record the past and present but not predict the future. If it were possible to add all of the depressive periods over the entire span of diabetes, that is from diagnosis to death, the percentage of patients suffering depression would be higher than the 20% in the survey.

Robinson, Fuller, and Edmeades worked with UK IDDM (Type I or Insulin Dependent Diabetes Mellitus) and NIDDM (Type II or Non-Insulin Dependent Diabetes Mellitus) adult blacks and whites. They found full depressive states in 8.5% of all and borderline depression in 19.2% of the Type I's and 14.6% of the Type II's. The presence of a depressed mental state did not correlate with sex, ethnic group, duration or type of diabetes, and social class but was significantly related to ability to cope, marital status, and amount of social contact. The advent of complications appeared to be important. There is a possibility that we have stumbled on a vicious cycle because depression may influence blood sugar control which may in turn cause complications (at least the short term ones of hypo- and hyperglycemia) thus leading to depression... Indeed, Lustman, Griffith, and Clouse tell of 5 year follow-up studies on a group of 37 diabetic adults with major depression. Of the 28 who were located at the end of 5 years, 18 had experienced a period of major depression within the previous 12 months. In a comparison group of nondepressed diabetic patients only 10% reported depression during the 5 years. Another group of Type I patients was found to consist of

25.9% women and 22.9% men who were depressed. However, this was a very special selection of diabetics because they were on a waiting list for pancreas transplants. Delving into the minds of people who want pancreas transplants is a whole other thing.

In a 1989 Weyerer's team, 3 groups of people were compared. They were normal healthy subjects, diabetic patients, and people with other physical illnesses. The 2 sick groups had about the same amount of psychological problems (significantly more than the normals) but in the diabetics this was due almost exclusively to depression while the other group suffered a variety of mental problems. Manic-depressives were examined for diabetes and found to have more (10%) than the general population (2%). Other psychiatric disorders also included more diabetics.

Mental condition is important as shown by Littlefield et al who studied social support given to 158 Type I diabetics between the ages of 17 and 78 years. Where functional impairment was present, depression was present but the degree was moderated by good social support. Even greater physical impairment could be stopped from causing depression with the presence of sufficient perceived support. The findings suggest that individuals with inadequate support are most at risk of becoming depressed when disability related to illness increases.

In assessing the effect of peripheral neuropathy on depression in 64 NIDDM women aged 55-74 years, Geringer and her group found the 12 depressed subjects had no greater neuropathy than the others. The authors make the interesting suggestion that the depression may be the result of an organic affective disorder. In other words, it could be the result of a central nervous system process that has parallel effects in the periphery (arms and legs) and in the emotions. Both would then be the result of the same physical mechanism.

Mentioned above was the possible effect of depression on blood sugar control. The effect of stress on such control is generally accepted but what is the effect of stress on depression? An Australian group discusses a 43 year old NIDDM man who was severely depressed and required insulin for blood glucose management. Treatment for depression caused his insulin requirements to lessen to the point where 3 months after beginning therapy he was free from the need for any medication for diabetes and had a normal glucose tolerance test. An intriguing story but only 1 case.

Many diabetic men are reported troubled by impotence. Both IDDM (22) and NIDDM (15) subjects were reported to suffer from generalized anxiety disorder and depression which probably contributed to their impotence as it does in nondiabetic males. Neuropathic problems played a part as well. Of insulin-treated diabetic women, 47% reported sexual dysfunction but their mental status was not reported. Still, when an important life drive is not satisfied, some depression must result.

For a self-caring diabetic, good blood sugar control is a strong concern. When depression was studied in its relationship to the appearance of diabetic symptoms (frequent urination, thirst, loss of weight) a correlation with glycosylated hemoglobin (a measure of glucose control over a period of several weeks) did not appear. What did show up was a relationship between hyperglycemic and hypoglycemic episodes and depression. Both may be life threatening circumstances whose possibility and presence are dealt with daily by the person taking insulin. They are to be avoided and their occurrence can cause depression.

Low and high blood sugars are short-term complications of diabetes and its treatment. Long-term complications can be mentally devastating. Loss of a leg hits hard. Some people give up and die. Some fight an inevitable amputation with all their strength, living through pain, minor surgery, infections - to try to keep the limb. But then, on the positive side, I remember an elderly black man already sightless, who said, after losing his leg and with a smile on his face, that he was going to keep enjoying his grandchildren, there was enough of him left for that. Many of the blind diabetics I know seem to be a happy, adjusted lot but still it comes out in conversation, that they are always aware of living with a loss and it depresses them. Even if vision loss is not total, the associated destruction of self-management skills can be disastrous. Think of the loss of independence when patients can no longer determine their own blood sugar levels or fill a syringe with the correct amount of insulin. Other daily living activities and self-sufficiency skills are gone as well. Of the 29 diabetics studied by Bernbaum, Albert, and Duckro, 16 had stable visual impairment (including total blindness) and 13 had fluctuating visual impairment. The first group was better compensated than the second, but all patients benefited from a rehabilitative intervention program as shown by significantly improved psychological profiles. Teaching ways around problems seems to help.

Indeed, education to enhance self-esteem and learn self-care benefited poorly informed and non-self-controlling diabetics. A week-long outpatient education program was participated in by 165 patients. The whole procedure was repeated at 6 months with 124 participants. Those who entered the program with high levels of emotional well-being or good self-care patterns tended to change little, if at all. People who entered the program with low levels of emotional well-being or with poor self-care patterns, improved substantially. A well-designed educational program can improve emotional status.

It should be noted that success can lift a mood. According to Friis and Nanjunappa, unemployment is associated with diabetes and employability problems are accompanied by higher depression levels among diabetic persons than among non-diabetic persons. They found employment to be the most significant predictor of a depressive state and suggest that special employment and counseling programs be available to diabetics with job troubles.

More difficult to help is the depressed husband of a chronically ill wife. The number of illness demands experienced by the man was a significant predictor of his levels of depression. This in turn affected the marital adjustments. Both illness demands and level of marital adjustment predicted coping behavior used. When illness demands and marital adjustment were high, introspection characterized by feedback, reflection and discussion was often seen. Incidentally, when this type of coping existed, father-child relationships were identified with more frequent interchanges. It makes sense. A person with better coping techniques, copes better.

Living with diabetes, as living with any chronic disease, is hard. While not a "Why me?" sayer, I do find myself thinking that I didn't expect to grow up to be like this. We feel all the losses - jobs, eyes, feeling in the feet, freedom to eat, feeling well, spontaneity in activities, indifference to our bodies, etc, etc. Sometimes the misfortunes are overwhelming. Depression sets in. The goal should be to make it short. Perhaps it serves a purpose.

The very expensive, huge Diabetes Control and Complications Trial altered American treatment of diabetes. The rate of eye and kidney complications was slowed by frequent blood sugar tests and multiple daily doses of insulin. Written in 1993, this column addresses the stresses imposed on diabetic individuals by a seemingly unqualified advance.

DCCT - Bad or Good

Medical journals are now carrying accounts of a huge experiment designed to prove that high blood sugar causes some of the major complications of diabetes. Retinopathy or eye disease, nephropathy or kidney disease, and neuropathy or nerve disease are the complications studied. It was named the DCCT which stands for Diabetes Control and Complications Trial. Over 1300 Type I (insulin dependent) diabetics attending 29 health care centers in America and Canada, took part. The experiment was stopped one year early because it was felt that enough data had been collected so that all diabetics should benefit from the results.

I wish the findings of the DCCT were more conclusive - 90% chance of no complications - but they aren't. Let me tell you about the study.

Half of those who participated cared for their disease in the old fashioned way. That is, they took insulin once or twice a day and measured blood sugar once a day. They were the control group. Patients in the experimental group administered insulin either in multiple (3 or more) injections or with an insulin pump which dispensed a constant flow of insulin with extra given at meal times or as needed. The goal of tight control is to keep blood sugar levels between 80 and 140 mg/dl except for a period of time after meals when the food is being digested. This group tested blood glucose a minimum of four times a day. Treating diabetes this way allows patients to try for tight control of their blood sugar levels. Physicians hope that tight control will avoid at least the microvascular complications of diabetes. Those are the complications we are talking about.

With tight control, retinopathy was reduced or slowed in 70% of patients under tight control - only 50% were referred to an eye surgeon for treatment and treated. Nephropathy - signalled by rising urinary protein - was reduced or slowed by 50%. Neuropathy showed a 60% decrease. There are however, side effects. Severe hypoglycemia - that's low blood sugar - occurred 3 times more frequently in people trying for tight control than in those using older approaches to insulin administration. Hypoglycemia can be quite dangerous. They also experienced periods of unconsciousness, probably due to the very low blood glucose.

Severe episodes of hypoglycemia (714) were reported by 216 patients. Of these, 77% were in intensively treated patients. 55% happened at night during sleep with 43% between midnight and 8 am. Of those occurring during the daytime, there were **no** warning symptoms in 36%. That's important to diabetics because hypoglycemia must be treated quickly. Going on with the results of the trial, patients liable to suffer severe hypoglycemia while trying for tight control, could be identified. They had a history of severe hypoglycemic incidents, longer duration of diabetes, higher baseline HbA_{1c} and a lower recent HbA1c. HbA1c is a measure of average blood sugar levels during the last 7-8 weeks.

The DCCT Research Group concluded that not every diabetic should be treated intensively. Those identified by predictive factors as being prone to severe hypoglycemia, should probably be eliminated from the study. In other words, individualized treatment. More data must be collected to determine which patients should try for tight control because the age range included in this experiment was narrow. Very few minority patients were included so watch out if you are black or Hispanic or something else. We already know that diabetes presents differently in different ethnic groups. Diabetes is not a uniform disease.

DCCT did not achieve *great* blood sugar control. What they got was average blood sugars of 155 mg/dl with HbA1cs of 7.2%.

Values in nondiabetic people are 110 mg/dl and 6.05%. Such differences are significant.

DCCT did achieve important weight gain with tight blood sugar control. There were attendant medical and mental problems. I suspect that both higher than desired blood sugar levels and weight gain may be due to a desire to avoid hypoglycemia. Eating more. Taking less insulin. We know that patients lie to their health care providers. It has been shown that they record more acceptable glucose levels than were measured by their meters. Why accept without question patient recorded values in this study. Hypoglycemia is frightening and, speaking for myself, I try desperately (if unsuccessfully) to avoid it.

We should also note that tight control is more costly than old fashioned control not only in terms of cash but also in terms of time. It's easy to say that doing a blood sugar takes only a few minutes but consider the time spent in having the equipment available (packing and carrying it when you're away from home). One increased money outlay is for the strips necessary to perform a blood sugar test. They cost approximately fifty American cents each. When the test is done four times a day the total is two dollars. You do the math. Multiply by 365 days a year.

****

Those are the facts. What follows are my opinions. I speak only for myself. But please remember, I am a Type I diabetic.

My intention is not to Pooh-Pooh an important study. My purpose is to look at the findings without rose colored glasses. DCCT results certainly show that good blood sugar control is a significant factor in reducing the number of Type I diabetics who will suffer major and costly complications of their disease. Remember, however, that not all diabetics are afflicted with these complications. Only about 40% of Type I diabetics get nephropathy according to Eli A. Friedman, MD. We can then say that 60% of insulin dependent diabetics do not have to take the risks involved in tight control with the purpose of protecting against kidney failure.

My point is that tight control can be dangerous. I fear teaching physicians to treat their patients in this way. Fear for several reasons. Unless emphasis is placed on screening patients, many will be put in jeopardy when they are taught to handle their blood sugars in an attempt to gain and maintain normal values. If left to endocrinologists perhaps it would be handled right but not all diabetics are seen by these specialists and primary care physicians may, understandably, not fully grasp what they are doing.

Note should be taken that a cross section of patients with insulin dependent diabetes was not used. Certain groups were not included. I can understand not wanting to work with noncompliant patients. Data from them would not be reliable. However, patients whose blood glucose was difficult to control were also left out.

What am I left with? There is a conclusion that high blood sugar is implicated as a significant factor in causing the three complications (eye, kidney, and nerve disease) which are thought to be due to pathology of minor blood vessels. But we must consider the figures. Still significant are the 30, 40, and 50% of diabetics who will have these complications. That's a lot of people.

Complications are expensive. Dialysis or kidney transplants cost thousands of dollars but tight control isn't cheap either. Hospitalizations, emergency room visits, and ambulance rides brought on by hypoglycemia are costly. I will mention again the interference with life necessitated by an attempt at tight control. As I sit and write at my computer I am always aware that I must stop, not at a good point in my work, but when the clock tells me to do a blood sugar.

O.K. Money isn't the only important factor. Can the goal be realized? Can the diabetic maintain euglycemia (normal blood sugar levels)? I can't and I'm a fairly compliant patient. When I've had three or four days of good control I cheer. I've done it. But then there are the times when I'm way low or way high with no explanation that I can find. That's the nature of the disease. If it were possible to predict what the blood sugar level is I wouldn't have to test for it. Diabetes is not a logical disease.

Now let me get to the reason why the DCCT results are the subject of this column.

Following a report in the May 22, 1993 issue of The Lancet, a distinguished British medial journal, The New York Times published (on May 23) an article interpreting it. Dr. Jay Skyler, a well known authority in the field and past president of the American Diabetes Association, was one of the people they correctly interviewed. His credentials are impeccable. Noting the increase in hypoglycemic episodes, even to loss of consciousness, he asserts that patients would choose this to impaired vision, end stage renal disease, and the pain and daily discomforts of neuropathy.

Dr. Skyler has probably never been unconscious on the floor for twelve hours. I have. I've also had a kidney transplant, vision loss (No - I'm not blind but there are big problems), and neuropathy keeps me in pain a good part of the time and seriously affects my digestive tract. I'm still scared silly by my time on the floor. Not only was twelve hours lost to me but days after when I wasn't functioning. I have no memory of my trip to the hospital. I've been told by the people who rescued me that they were there but you sure can't prove it by my recollections. A piece of my life is gone. I was out of control. Result: when I think there is a possibility of "going out" again I eat a lot making good blood sugar control impossible. I also choose to try for blood sugar values not in the recommended 80-140 mg/dl range but at a 150-180 mg/dl spread.

Which would I choose - complications or extreme hypoglycemia? Hard decision. Selecting the better of two "bads" is difficult. At this point in my life I would select the possibility of complications. Others may, and should, choose for themselves. Tight control is obviously good and certainly, if the diabetic selects a path aiming at less than perfect control, the outcome will be more beneficial than no control.

I have a wonder. Maybe if tight control was begun when the diagnosis of diabetes was made, or even before when the appropriate circulating antibody levels indicate a strong possibility of developing symptomatic diabetes and blood sugar amounts become higher than normal, perhaps the rate of reduction of complications might approach 100%. If the cause of minor vessel complications is high blood sugar, Type II (Non-Insulin Dependent Diabetes Mellitus) must also be brought under good control. Extending my argument for early good control is the problem of knowing when Type II diabetes begins (thought to be 7-12 years before diagnosis) arises. Frequent screening of populations believed prone to diabetes - native Americans, Hispanics, etc. - should find Type IIs at the start of their disease and maybe avoid these complications which they share with Type Is.

Before I close there is another thought. It was only after diabetes could be treated with newly discovered insulin that diabetics lived long enough to develop complications. There is no great experience with *compliant* patients *who have many incidents of hypoglycemia*. What may this cause?

My message is: Be careful. Nonconclusive DCCT results may be applied with bad results.

Barry's superb sense of humor is illustrated by the title of this 1992 column that returned to the diabetic foot but also recognized the threat of systemic joint and bone disease in diabetes. She closes with an emblematic clarion call that infused others with her life force: "Persist, Persist, Persist."

...Knee Bone Connected to the Thigh Bone, Thigh Bone Connected to the Hip Bone...

Of course, with diabetics, who are all mixed up anyway, you feel like singing: knee bone connected to the skull bone...

Bones, like every other part of the body, are affected by diabetes thus there is no reason to expect bones to be excluded from this involvement and indeed they are not. Charcot joint, osteomyelitis, osteoporosis, and arthritic diseases as well as the bone disease of dialysis, and limb amputation in transplant recipients occur in both types of diabetes - that is IDDM (Type I or Insulin Dependent Diabetes Mellitus) and NIDDM (Type II or Non-Insulin Dependent Diabetes Mellitus). When the question "Why?" is posed it must be answered with the standard response to the "whys?" of diabetic complications - nobody knows for sure.

In the case of Charcot joint, many believe that the combination of diabetic neuropathy and painless trauma causes dislocation and collapse of the tarsal (ankle and foot) joints. The resulting pathology of the soft tissues and bone can appear as if they were due to infection. Proper care depends on correct diagnosis. Surgery may be recommended. Long term treatment is best placed in the hands of a podiatrist familiar with diabetes. Spotting quietly developing Charcot joint is one of many reasons why physicians should examine the feet of their diabetic patients at every visit. Early detection may result in shifting the patient to wearing proper shoes and a chance of preventing later limb loss.

Troubled diabetic feet can be classified into: 1. neuropathic (caused by nerve damage) feet showing ulcers, 2. Charcot joint (with edema and good blood flow), and 3 feet with bad circulation and an absence of pulses. Neuropathic foot ulcers may occur where the blood vessels are stiff and dilated as a result of calcification. Realize that if the walls of blood vessels are coated with a cement-like substance containing calcium they cannot contract and relax. When the foot can't feel and small bones have shifted, a new pattern of weight bearing can develop. Natural adjustment of foot placement on the floor does not occur and constant application of pressure on one spot is the result. Ulcers usually develop under calluses such as those that occur on the ball of the foot and are best prevented from occurring or recurring by the ministrations of a podiatrist or chiropodist. Molded insoles which redistribute weight on the foot may be called for. Neuropathy prevents a person from feeling how the body's weight is pressing on one point, a sensation which causes normal people to frequently shift slightly. Constant force on one point causes breakdown of the tissue resulting in an ulcer. Infection may set in and slow or absent healing becomes a problem.

Charcot joint is often preceded by broken foot and ankle bones and can develop rapidly but more about that later. Nerve caused edema can be treated successfully in 72% of the cases (Edmonds, M.E, 1986).

An assortment of neurologic disorders may produce damage to the foot but diabetes mellitus is the most common cause. Various radiography techniques are used to tell if infection is present and if it extends from soft tissue to bone. There is a report of Charcot joint appearing as acute osteomyelitis which is bacterial bone infection.

Nerve damage of joints was first described in 1831 by Mitchel but it wasn't until 1868 that Charcot noted destructive joint changes and remarked on both the clinical findings and the mechanisms which he thought caused it. It is interesting to recognize that the first joint which got his attention, was a knee and the condition was believed to be associated with syphilis. Charcot joint is thought of as a slowly progressive, chronic, degenerative form of joint deterioration characterized by bone absorption and multiple fractures but Slowman, Braunstein, and Brandt speak of 3 patients with long standing IDDM who developed joint deterioration within weeks of minor foot or ankle trauma. It has not been possible to duplicate Charcot joint in lab animals so it is hard to study. Edelman et al in 1987, writing in the Archives of Internal Medicine, assert that trauma is secondary to neuropathy in Charcot joint development. A neurally initiated vascular reflex can lead to increased blood flow (in other words too much blood and higher blood pressure in the foot and ankle due to nerve damage in the blood vessels). Earlier, 1980, Kristiansen wrote in a Scandinavian journal, that foot fractures, even minor ones, must be carefully treated by eliminating weight-bearing to avoid joint degeneration.

A major problem in diagnosing Charcot joint is telling the difference between bone infection and nerve caused joint disease. Three x-ray-like techniques are used. Bone scans came first and are of limited value. Magnetic resonance imaging (MRI) was used on 14 diabetic patients. Understanding that infection is often present in more than one site, MRI evaluation showed 8 cases of bone infection (osteomyelitis), 7 abscesses (tissue infection), 5 nerve caused joint problems, 4 septic arthritis conditions (painful joints), and 4 tendon sheath inflammations. Clinical or surgical/pathological confirmation of all but 9 of these diagnoses was made, resulting in an evaluation of MRI as a good way to classify the troubled diabetic foot. Scintigraphy (use of a special camera to get images after giving radioactive substances) gave false positive infection results for 3 patients while Indium labelled white cell imaging gave correct results on those 3 patients. Searching out Indium labelled white cells is a good, while not perfect, method of telling infection from nerve caused bone pathology.

It is interesting to note that Charcot joint is not always a foot and ankle problem. Occurrence in the upper extremities of diabetics is reported, with bone resorption and multiple fractures described in the shoulder. A single case of Charcot joint of the spine has been published.

The importance of correctly differentiating infection from Charcot joint can be emphasized by telling what happens if they are not told apart. Untreated infection can lead to amputation and ignored bone pathology can go on to deformity. A high index of suspicion is the best way to avoid complications. Diabetic patients with long standing neuropathy, who present with warm, swollen, red feet and no signs or symptoms of infection, must be considered to be suffering from Charcot joint. Initial treatment consists of complete abstinence from weight bearing. Only after swelling, warmth, and redness disappear can the use of protective weight bearing methods be considered.

Bone infections are sometimes difficult to stop. First, a determination of whether the infection is confined to soft tissue or involves bone, must be made. Foot ulcers may be deep enough to expose tendons and bone; it can be assumed when this is the case, that infection extends into the bone. Radiographic techniques which diagnosis the condition can be used to judge how far the debridement (surgical cleaning of the area) should extend. Sometimes these bacteria caused wound problems don't heal well and the use of hyperbaric oxygen therapy can be tried. Using such a device raises the amount of oxygen in the immediate environment and may stimulate wound healing.

Osteoporosis is not an infection but rather describes poor bones which in their thinness and lack of strength, are apt to break easily. You know that all the cells of the body are periodically replaced by new ones. It seems that in diabetes (IDDM and NIDDM) there is a low turnover of bone cells. Working with diabetic rats, Verhaeghe's group showed slow formation of bone cells while the relative percent of calcium remained the same as in normal animals. Shao, Wang, Hu, and Zhang examined 11 IDDM humans and 19 NIDDM humans as well as controls. Calcium, potassium, and x-ray investigations were similar in all three groups. Type I patients showed increased serum levels of parathyroid hormone and AKP. Changes in calcium activity in diabetic rats was reported by Verhaeghe et al. Urinary calcium excretion was increased 10-fold and active intestinal absorption of calcium was completely abolished. Vitamin D action was also markedly decreased. According to Saggesse et al., the increased parathyroid hormone may account for lowering the magnesium level which shows in the decreased bone mineral content in 29 children with IDDM. No matter how you look at it, damage is common in the bones of diabetics.

A lack of bone cell formation and turnover is present in diabetic rats as well as diabetic humans. Tetracycline remedies the condition in rats seeming to correct both the metabolism and morphology of bone cell precursors.

We have seen then, that weak bones in diabetes can be caused by either the lack of production of good dense bone or resorption of the existing bone. In general, hormone related disease has a bad effect on the skeleton. In children, disturbances are common in growth and maturation. In adults bone damage is manifested as the result of altered bone maintenance and metabolism. The child often presents as short and suffering from generalized osteoporosis. Older patients have generalized osteoporosis particularly if they are not obese. Calcification of interdigital arteries of the foot are common. Cimmino and Cutolo report that fasting blood sugars of patients with osteoarthritis were significantly higher than those in controls. They evaluated 1026 patients, 56 of whom had diabetes. Hyperglycemic osteoarthritic patients had greater pain at rest. That development of bone degenerative disease is related to high blood sugar is concluded by the authors.

1983 produced an account noting a prevalence of Type I diabetes in the close relatives of patients with rheumatoid arthritis. In 13% (39) of 295 patients with classical or definite rheumatoid arthritis, a first or second degree relative with Type I diabetes was present and 13% (38) had a close relative with autoimmune thyroid disease. There is then the possibility of a common genetic mechanism producing both diseases.

People with end stage renal disease treated with hemodialysis and who suffered from diabetes showed a lower bone mineral density than non-diabetic patients.

All the bones connected to each other seem to be in poor condition but we keep walking or hobbling along with enough strength in our hands to do blood sugars and inject insulin or swallow pills. Bone disease is not a good complication of diabetes but at least it's usually not life threatening. Persist. Persist. Persist.

For stark reality, this brutally frank head on confrontation with body damage in diabetes may be more than many newly diagnosed diabetic individuals wish to hear. On the other hand, physicians shy away from preparing their patients for the bowel, bladder, and vascular complications that lie ahead. Typical of Barry's hand holding is her concluding admonition in this 1990 column lending support and encouragement.

The Physical Side of Diabetes

The handicaps don't always show, but they're there. People react differently to the appearance, in themselves, of limitations. Some cope. Some don't. There is hope for those who try and they may be successful in living with their infirmities. "Why me?", is not the question they ask. "That's the way the cookie crumbles.", is their reaction. Difficult adjustments must be made. Accepting the fact that you are handicapped is not easy. Now all the disabling side effects reported on here, don't happen to all diabetics. A certain percentage of patients live without suffering bad consequences but they are not the ones I am talking about.

Since the whole body can be involved, my problem is where to start discussing the physical effects of diabetes. The highest point is the head. I'll begin there.

Right under the hair and scalp and skull is the brain, the site for strokes. Cerebrovascular accidents, that is hemorrhages or clots in the vessels, can have mild or devastating effects. The result is that the brain finds new nerve paths to accomplish tasks it has lost the ability to direct. For instance, nerve impulses controlling muscle manipulation to write, need to discover different pathways in the brain. Retraining strength in the hand requires stimulation. Squeezing a special device or a roll of socks can help accomplish this. Walking can be interfered with. Intelligible speech can disappear. Stroke is a handicap that shows, at least at first. Its effects can be encouraged to disappear. I knew a man who had had a severe stroke. He spoke only a few words to me and they were not clear but English was not his native tongue. As an elected official the time came for him to run for office again and he made political speeches. I didn't hear him, and I wouldn't have understood his language if I had, but people told me that he spoke well and understandably. Re-election was his goal and he won. Much work with speech and other therapists enabled him to succeed. Effort was the key to his mastery of a hard set of circumstances.

A condition that also shows, is blindness. A cane or Seeing Eye dog should be obvious to the sighted indicating that a person has a problem. I won't say: "Close your eyes for an hour and see what it is like." because that will not simulate blindness but only the new condition. Training is available and usually quickly given to those whose ability to see is lost. Some of them take advantage. Some don't. I remember two young people who lost sight at approximately the same time. Three years later, one had a cane and a seeing eye dog, used public transportation, had returned to school and was on his way to graduating, he was learning the computer, and was looking for a girl to date (found one, too). The second lived in a wheel chair and was incapable of getting herself a glass of water in her own home. She lived with a full time companion. Think about these two.

Problems that most of us have never even considered, like finding the right elevator button to push, exist for the sightless. Selecting the right bill or correct coin are all predicaments that can be overcome. And there are others. Once I was about to enter a room where four young blind men whom I knew, were having a discussion. After I heard the subject, I turned around quietly and left. Their serious conversation was on how to hit the urinal (which was a matter of triumph anyway, since they all had kidney transplants). The blind who manage can do many activities. They cook, they work, use public transportation, raise children, ski, do carpentry, do self-monitoring of blood glucose, and smile.

But not everyone who loses vision, loses all. Degrees between just a little trouble seeing to well beyond the state of "legally blind", arise. Such situations do not show in the big, outside world; strangers don't make accommodations for you. For instance, when you are taking a long time at the cashier trying to tell one coin from another, and people behind you get impatient, they just don't know your state. Those who succeed in living with a loss of sight are probably creative and have a sense of humor. I know a daughter who told her mother that if Mama didn't do what daughter wanted, daughter would get up in the middle of the night and move the furniture around. Mama laughed. Another woman comes to mind. She must have cornered the market in red nail polish. Everything got marked. The oven dial was easy for her to find but the correct setting was not, so she marked 350 in bright red, etc., etc. The outside world can be harder. If you can't read traffic lights, or see vehicles coming, you have the choice of sitting home or learning to cross the street when other people do. Attitude, wanting to do, helps people get done what they want to get done.

That doesn't mean that the problems don't exist. They certainly do and some are harder to live with than others. Gastrointestinal problems fall into both categories. Delayed stomach emptying and slow moving of the food through the digestive tract is uncomfortable and makes blood sugar control difficult. The dilemma can usually be handled with medication. Diabetic diarrhea, on the other hand, is very difficult to manage and seldom responds to treatment. This type of diarrhea is not the kind that most people occasionally face. Usually nocturnal, it is rapid, massive, and accompanied by a loss of sphincter control resulting in soiled beds. The outcome is a very unpleasant predicament. After the first episode, whose approach was not predicted, the use of adult diapers can help but it remains a more than distasteful circumstance.

Bladder dysfunction is not as messy but certainly is a physical consequence of diabetes. Most people who suffer bladder troubles and who need to, can learn self-catheterization and take care of themselves in the privacy of the bathroom. The outside world need never know.

Another thing strangers may not be aware of, is the successful use of an artificial leg. Some amputees limp, others don't but that holds true for nonamputees as well. Some people cope beautifully. An old black man of my acquaintance comes to mind. I only mention that he was black so you will know he had been coping all his life. When I visited him in the hospital after they had just removed his leg, he greeted me with a warm smile, even though his blindness kept him from seeing me, and said: "There's plenty of me left to enjoy my granddaughter who loves me, and my friends." And then he laughed. Contrast this with a woman of equal years who lay moaning in a darkened room after her amputation. "I don't want to see or hold it." she said of her newly born grandchild. She never walked again. But a friend of mine, a double amputee, legally blind, walked into an Italian restaurant so she could eat her favorite meal. What a personal triumph!

I knew two other double amputees, neither confined to a wheelchair. The older of the pair gardened and climbed ladders to paint his house. He had the joy of playing with his grandchildren. The second, was a drunk. Don't laugh. He was successful in what he chose to do. Then there was the man who lost one leg but didn't want to accept government handouts. Child care, including walking down three flights of steps to take the kids to the school bus and picking them up again, became his task so his wife could work and earn their daily bread. A man to be admired.

As you can see, I have great respect for people who live cheerfully with their infirmities.

Even if legs and fingers aren't removed, they can be troublesome. Foot neuropathy doesn't show but it can cause difficulties such as bruising from bumping into obstacles or stepping on objects. Diabetic neuropathy can cause feet not to shift to distribute weight more equitably, thus resulting in a lot of pressure being applied to one spot on the sole of the foot. That can cause the formation of an ulcer. Diabetic foot ulcers heal slowly and not at all if the patient is unaware of them (no sensation due to neuropathy leads to ignorance of their existence) and doesn't treat them correctly. Neuropathy in another form can lead to Charcot's joint (deformation and destruction of the ankle) which necessitates the wearing of a brace. A friend of mine, a young lady, has completely given up skirts and dresses. She wears slacks for everyday and special occasions to hide her braces. With a smile on her face, she carries it off beautifully.

Pins and needles and loss of sensation in the hands can lead women to dress less beautifully. When earring backs and necklace clasps become hard to manage, you can either give up jewelry or go to snap on ear baubles and long, slip over the head, strands. More serious is the presence of sensory neuropathy in the blind who may lose the ability to read braille. Probably other situations that I am not aware of, exist.

I do know, however, about the loss of kidney function due to diabetes. Renal failure was left for last in this report because *Renal Family* is a kidney patient's magazine. Before speaking about replacement therapies for failed kidneys, the uremic state should be mentioned. As with untreated diabetes, fatigue can be a major symptom. Constant exhaustion is not only debilitating but difficult to live with. A complaint such as this can generate a lack of sympathy from family and friends. At least a pain seems more real, more worthy of pity, than a vague: "I'm tired". "I can't climb those two steps.", receives about an equal amount of understanding. "Do your legs hurt"? "No". "Are they weak"? "No". "Well, what then"? "I don't know. I can't explain it". And so you crawl those stairs with noncommiserating help. Nowadays, when doctors don't allow patients to get as sick as they did years ago, these signs may not have shown up. Lucky patients, although they may not think so when faced with making a choice between available treatments. Other techniques for coping with renal shutdown exist but the three most common are: kidney transplantation, hemodialysis, and CAPD (Continuous Ambulatory Peritoneal Dialysis). The one that you can live with without daily physical involvement is transplantation. Hemodialysis, when done in a center, requires patient transportation to that center, usually three times a week. Because schedules are involved, daily activities may be interfered with and make holding a job hard. There is a very restrictive diet to follow. Both home cooking and restaurant meals become laborious in terms of compliance. More confining still, are the limitations on fluid intake. Food and drink regulations can take away from the pleasure of a social gathering. One may not always want to be treated specially. Extra care must be given to the site where the dialysis needles are implanted. The location must be protected from physical harm. And then there is the very substantial act of inserting, or having inserted, large needles into your arm. That's a difficult maneuver to cope with emotionally, yet in order to live on hemodialysis, it is necessary and so people contend. CAPD requires changing of fluid from bags, into and out of the abdominal cavity. CAPD involves a catheter and a sloshing. The catheter allows the fluid exchange but necessitates great care in its cleanliness and causes worries about things like your sex life, which need not be stopped. Sloshing refers to the fact that the patient walks around with a lot of fluid in his abdomen. I must admit I don't know how much noise is generated but a change in shape is obvious. Another physical thing to deal with.

Many bodily side effects of diabetes exist. The problem is - how to cope. No matter what the predicament, techniques of surmounting it are basically the same. A positive attitude, knowing that there are other people worse off, a desire to try to overcome, and a sense of humor are all invaluable. A loving, helpful, understanding, "significant others" group is too.

When you are faced with a dilemma, remember, others have made it. You can as well.

How Barry became preoccupied with the liver, lungs, and lymphatics in diabetes is revealed in this 1993 column that directly interprets science for the nonscientific diabetic patient. After reading transplant pioneer Thomas Starzl's autobiographical book, The Puzzle People, Barry sought further explanation of what the liver does or fails to do in the diabetic individual. Illustrating her quest for accuracy, Barry wrote Starzl and includes his reply as a source.

The "L" words. Liver, Lungs, Lymphatics

My 7 year old daughter was taught the following with the hope that it would help her correctly pronounce the "L" sound.

The one "L" lama, he's a priest.
The two "L" llama, he's a beast.
And I will bet a silk pajama, there isn't any three "L" lllama.

Don't take that bet.

We're going to find out about three "Ls" - liver, lungs, and lymphatics - and diabetes. Knowing nothing about my subjects before starting, I got a good education. Now it's your turn.

The gifted surgical researcher whose team is currently involved in baboon-to-man liver transplants, Thomas Starzl, has just published his autobiography, The Puzzle People (University of Pittsburgh Press; Pittsburgh, PA 15260 - American $24.95). I was fascinated with Starzl's repeated stress that insulin whose hormone action is important all through the body, must first go through the liver to maintain the health of that organ. My mind turned with questions: What do the livers of Type I diabetics who lack their own insulin and inject manufactured insulin into arms and legs far from the liver, look like? What do the livers of untreated Type I diabetics look like? How about the livers of pancreas transplant patients? Are their blood streams hooked up to the liver circulation somehow? I wrote. Starzl's answer came: We try to put the pancreas circulation upstream of the liver circulation...My other questions remained unanswered.

So, undaunted, I turned to the textbooks. Wouldn't it be nice if things were simple? The body works with carbohydrates, proteins, and lipids or fats. My mind said: Goody. I'll have 3 divisions - liver and carbohydrate, liver and protein, and liver and lipid. Ha! They're all connected. O.K. Jump in. Start with liver and carbohydrate.

Diabetics have messed up carbohydrate metabolism so lets begin by looking at normal metabolism. When carbohydrate is eaten, the mouth and stomach work together and change it into glucose (a simple sugar). Glucose goes from the intestine into the portal circulation - that's liver circulation. Eventually the glucose gets to the pancreas where beta cells in the Islets of Langerhans (special groups of cells) sense it and secrete insulin to lower the sugar level. However, at the same time, alpha cells (another special group of cells in the Islets of Langerhans of the pancreas) secrete a second hormone, glucagon, which raises blood sugar. Both hormones enter the vein leaving the pancreas and go to the next organ, the liver.

The liver has 2 ways to regulate blood sugar levels. First, it can make glucose. Second, it can break down glycogen which is stored glucose. (Glucose is stored as glycogen in muscles, too.) Insulin inhibits the formation of glucose and the breakdown of liver glycogen thus lowering blood sugar levels. Glucagon does just the opposite. The presence of both hormones, insulin and glucagon, controls the blood sugar level depending on the proportions of glucagon and insulin. Therefore, in diabetics where there is either not enough insulin or insulin that doesn't work right, more glucose is formed and more liver glycogen is broken down to glucose. Result: high blood sugar levels.

Don't breathe a sigh of relief and think: That's the end of liver and carbohydrate. No way. With a lot of extra glucose around, the liver gets busy and makes fatty acids out of it. When insulin is present, the fatty acids change into triglycerides which the circulatory system takes to the fat cells - adipocytes. Diabetics often have high triglyceride levels which may explain the high rate of coronary artery disease and strokes which go along with the disease. Most of these triglycerides come from the diet. Triglycerides as VLDL (very low density lipoproteins) are either put into the circulation or broken down in the liver, to LDL (low density lipoprotein) which is rich in cholesterol. Anything which uses up the body's available glucose will put the stored fatty acids back into circulation and cause them to be burned for fuel. Glucose is the important fuel for living things but when there is none, or when, as in the diabetic lack of insulin, it can't get into the cells, they look for fatty acids. Burned fatty acids become ketones. Beta cells don't respond to ketones until their level is very high. Then beta cells secrete insulin which would stop this process. If there are no beta cells, as in Type I or insulin dependent diabetes, insulin can't be secreted. Ketones are bad because they make the blood acidic. pH is the measure of acid and it must be kept very close to a fixed point of 7.4 to maintain life. Ketones then, are bad and good. At first, when no glucose is available, the brain and other tissues, burn them to keep alive. When too much ketone accumulates, the life of the whole being is threatened by changing pH.

Ketones have another function. They keep muscle cells from breaking down and burning protein when the supply of glucose is low or exhausted. That's important because muscle mass must be kept and because hormones and enzymes - which make possible the chemical reactions of the body - are also proteins and very vital ones. Insulin is a hormone and therefore, a protein. Diabetics make less protein than normal people and break down more. Insulin corrects this - at least in muscles. Livers make many proteins including those that are kept within its cells and those which are secreted - mostly as albumin. Diabetics make less protein to be secreted but not less of the other kind. Breakdown of protein in the liver happens in two different places inside the liver cells and is increased in diabetics. Breakdown just happens inside the fluid of the cell or it happens inside a structure in the cell called a lysosome. Insulin stabilizes lysosome membranes so we can assume diabetes weakens them.

Diabetes and the liver - not an easy tale.

However, have faith, our next subject is easier. Well, maybe not. It's easier for our minds because little is known about the lymphatic system and diabetes. It may not be easy for our diabetic bodies because things may be happening. I base that statement on my belief that diabetes affects every part of our carcasses. The right people just haven't looked yet.

For the future know a little about the lymphatic system. Unlike the blood circulation, it is not a closed system. There is a beginning (the littlest capillaries begin in the spaces between cells) and an end (the 2 large vessels - the thoracic duct on the left side and lower half of the body and the right duct both of which empty into the blood system on either side of the neck). The fluid or lymph is much like blood plasma but contains few cell; usually only lymphocytes. The lymphatic system has been described as a scavenger system draining the space between cells and removing things too big to enter the blood capillaries.

My other "L" organ is the lungs. I can't find information relating to diabetes and lungs. Again I'll say that I'm sure there must be some damage done by our disease but it hasn't been found yet.

Do you think I'm wrong? Should I change my mind and not be so dogmatic about diabetes and its effect on all parts of our bodies?

In 1992, concerned with dry and itching skin and having undergone surgical removal of skin growths thought to have malignant potential, Barry confronted the new challenge directly. Following library research, interviews with skin specialists (dermatologists) and much thought, Barry decided to share her findings and insights with Renal Family readers.

Skin

Skin: The external covering or integument of an animal body, esp. when soft and flexible.
The Living Webster Encyclopedic Dictionary of the English Language (1974)

Yup - that's what it is and we each have one. I didn't think I had any but the normal interactions with mine - an occasional cut, burn, or blemish. Then I noticed a growth. Removed. Sent to the pathologist. Report returned. Possible skin cancer. Surgeon goes a little deeper and into normal skin and sews me up. New pathology report: normal tissue. My private oncologist (my baby daughter specializes in cancers) tells me that even if it was a squamous cell carcinoma, there is nothing to worry about. I don't anyway. I'm not a worrier. The result, however, was to make this topic a little more fascinating to me, a little more personal. Why did I get this thing? Probably because I’m immunosuppressed to keep my kidney transplant but did having diabetes play any role?

As I've said before, diabetes is a disease that affects all parts of the body so there is no surprise in finding out that the skin is involved, too. None of the readings for this column mention skin growths and diabetes while immunosuppressive drugs are known to encourage tumors. My conclusion, then, is that the diabetes was not the cause of my problem (this time) but, boy, are there possibilities for the skin to be affected.

Goodfield and Millard writing from Notingham, UK, state rather bluntly that 100% of diabetic patients have skin involvement. During my first perusal of the literature all the skin conditions associated with diabetes seemed to fall into 2 categories: purely mechanical ones and those with an autoimmune basis.

Because I started off with a mention of immunosuppressive drugs, let me stay with immunology. IDDM (Type I or Insulin Dependent Diabetes Mellitus) people have an autoimmune condition. The body's killer lymphocytes (white blood cells) and antibodies attack (reject) a part of itself as though it was foreign tissue. Insulin producing Islet of Langerhans cells in the pancreas are the rejected pieces. When these cells are damaged lack of insulin leads to high blood sugar. NIDDMs (Type II or Non-Insulin Dependent Diabetes Mellitus) do not share the same reason for high blood sugars. Because of the way the researchers record their subjects, not always categorizing them, it is not always possible to determine if skin conditions affect IDDMs and NIDDMs differently.

A description by Abraham et al. of one diabetic patient who had psoriasis, necrobiosis lipoidica diabeticorum, granuloma annulare, vitiligo, with a history of recurrent erysipelas and mycotic infections (don't get scared - you'll soon know what all those things are) included the notation that there were both phenotypic (how something looks because of its inheritance - blue eyes, tall, cell characteristics) and functional defects in the cellular immunity (how white blood cells react) of the patient. This person's diabetic type was not specified. Regarding the psoriasis which is characterized by red spots covered with scales, Italian workers (Binazzi, Calandra, and Lisi) find highly significant correlation in the occurrence of diabetes with psoriasis. The relationship is strongest in patients under 50 years of age and male.

One report exists of a rare patient. To start with, she is a Japanese Type I diabetic - few Type Is exist in her country. Add to that her affliction with idiopathic thrombocytic purpura (bleeding into the skin producing purplish skin and a low platelet count with no known cause). She and her parents had Grave's disease (a large hyperactive thyroid as in President Bush). Her mother shared with her the most common genetic types found in Japanese IDDMs. There is mention in another paper of a patient with Grave's disease and skin problems. Is there a connection?

Less unique is the appearance of Vitiligo in IDDMs. Diminished or absent function of melanocytes (skin cells that contain the pigment melanin) causes spotty loss of pigmentation particularly on the extremities. The condition has no symptoms but can be emotionally troubling to people with darker skin. Vitiligo has been reported in both major kinds of diabetes but most consider it more highly associated with IDDM. Macaron et al. studied 5 children with vitiligo and found that 4 of the 5 had thyroid, adrenal or gastric antibodies. In 2 of the children the skin disorder preceded the appearance of diabetes. HLA (gene categories) types associated with IDDM were present in 3 of the children. All these facts point to an autoimmune cause and indeed, Fairfax and Leatham associate idiopathic heart block (electrical communication between the heart chambers not working right and due to an unknown cause) with autoimmune diseases notably diabetes, Grave's disease, vitiligo, etc..

Associating a second disorder with diabetes can be tricky but try this one. In 557 patients with granuloma annulare (usually on the front and sides of the arms and legs of children and young adults, without symptoms, appears as a slightly raised, flat topped, ring shaped, flesh colored, lesion) Muhlemann and Williams found 16 Type I diabetics. They only expected 0.9, O.K. that could be due to high blood sugar or other characteristics of diabetes but 2 more of the 557 developed Type I diabetes within 5 years.

A disease that often appears before the onset of diabetes - like a marker of signal - is acanthosis nigricans. Characterized by thickening and darkening of the skin on the neck and in the armpits, it is associated with Type II diabetes. Acanthosis nigricans is seen in 2 classes of patients both of whom are highly insulin resistant (takes a lot of extra insulin to lower blood sugar). The first consists of young women who show male traits such as hairiness, and the second consists of older women (rarely men) who have features of autoimmune disease.

That covers all the known skin conditions that are obviously mixed up with immunity. Future research may show more mechanisms that fit the pattern.

*****

Scleredema diabeticorum is a common (2.5% of diabetics) and distinct skin manifestation of diabetes. Thickening of the skin on the neck and back -a second condition in which the skin thickens on the back **** why? oh why? oh why? - which causes discomfort when it no longer bends easily. In general, skin thickness is increased in insulin dependent diabetes and correlates with the duration of the diabetes. Of 100 hospital-based diabetics in a study done by Satar et al., 14 had scleredema diabeticorum. More retinopathy and albuminuria was present in the 14 than in the others. Duration of the skin disease correlated with the duration of the diabetes. Cole, Headley, and Skowsky diagnosed 17 patients with scleredema diabeticorum and classify 15 of them as Type II diabetics. Another group of workers (Toyota et al.) report its occurrence in insulin dependant obese patients but my thought is that they may be insulin <u>treated</u> Type IIs. There are other categories of scleredema but diabeticorum is specific for diabetics and is one of many skin lesions specific for diabetes.

Current interest in the effect of glucose on collagen may unravel the mystery as the collagen changes to a stiff new form in the prolonged presence of hyperglycemia.

Bullosis diabeticorum - blisters to us lay people - is another such lesion. These little guys look like burn blisters, occur on the feet or hands, disappear by themselves and often recur. Males with long standing diabetes are usually the victims. Like scleredema, the cause is unknown but microscopic examination shows blister formation between 2 skin layers thus explaining the lack of scar formation when they heal.

Young adult white women are most commonly afflicted with necrobiosis lipoidica diabeticorum which appears as brown patches on the fronts of the legs. When they ulcerate protection from injury is necessary. Usually a loss of feeling is present in the lesion. Biopsies of the areas characteristically show thickening of the blood vessel walls and sometimes occlusion. Several treatments exist including surgery.

Now here's a colorful condition. Purpura. Following edema of the legs, small red spots which are leakage of a small amount of blood, turn into small pigmented spots. Purpura, pigmentation, red toes, and yellow nails could occur together. (No comment.)

Skin diseases are important to physicians and the diseases that occur mainly in diabetics (necrobiosis lipoidica diabeticorum, blisters of unknown origin, granuloma annulare, etc.) but which may appear before the diabetes should alert doctors to a possible diagnosis of diabetes. Easy to see and easy to study, skin can be used to learn about the pathology of diabetes.

An easy thing to examine is blood flow in the forearm. Tur, Vosipovitch, and Bar did just that in 25 Type II diabetics and 25 control subjects. They found microcirculatory changes associated with advanced retinopathy. Retinopathy is capillary disease in the retina of the eye. Katz and his group looked closely at capillaries of Type II diabetics and determined that when increased blood flow was required normal people used more capillaries and diabetics increased the flow in each capillary. Capillary density and the number of endothelial cells in vessel walls had little to do with the changes in blood flow and were only slightly involved with altered permeability. The same increased blood flow pattern was present in patients with successful kidney-pancreas transplants.

More skin problems develop in people with working organ transplants due to the immunosuppressive drugs they take which alter their immune systems. Diabetics are not exempted from these circumstances but I will not discuss that aspect of diabetic skin disease here. Indeed, so much information exists about diabetic skin that I do not have room to discuss it all in the space allotted for my column. More next issue.

Continuing her inquiry into why diabetes is associated with skin disorders, Barry in 1992 aptly summarizes a complex medical literature. Lucid, at the lay level, and spiked with humor, this column well portrays Barry's strengths as a medical communicator.

More About Diabetic Skin

Skin blood flow is reduced in diabetics and results in a deficient response when the body has need to increase blood flow. Normal people use more capillaries. Diabetics make the vessels in use work harder individually. Fewer capillaries exist in the skin of diabetics accounting for such a reaction.

Blood flow patterns in the hands of diabetic men were investigated by Hauer et al. who determined skin blood flow and then immersed the right hands of 34 diabetic men (and 12 nondiabetic controls) in ice water. Measurements are deduced based on the temperature of the hands. Recovery from immersion was abnormally slow in the diabetics. Severe autonomic neuropathy correlated with these findings leading to the thought that heat reflex regulation may be controlled by the autonomic nervous system. Chan, MacFarlane, and Bowsher studied feet of 35 diabetics with painful neuropathy (33 controls). Skin temperature was higher than normal over the weight-bearing parts of the foot - ball and heel. Pain was not affected by changes in temperature of the skin. No help to people with painful neuropathy but more proof that skin blood flow changes with diabetes. Skin oxygen pressure in 3 groups of people was measured by Gaylarde and coworkers. Controls, diabetics without neuropathy (12), and diabetics with neuropathy (9) comprised the study groups. Higher skin oxygen pressure was found in diabetics with neuropathy. In the first 2 sets the oxygen pressure was greater in the legs than in the feet but there was no leg-to-foot difference when neuropathy was present. A lack of vasodilatory response in the patients with neuropathy may contribute to their nonhealing ulcers, protracted infections, and gangrene.

Skin blood flow changes and the observation that to increase the flow no more capillaries are called into play but that each vessel tries harder, may be explained by the comment that diabetic skin has fewer capillaries than normal. A histological (microscopic) picture of diabetic skin was obtained by Braverman and his colleagues when they biopsied the buttocks (ouch !) of 15 patients with long standing Type I diabetes. Pericytes and endothelial cells are cells structuring capillaries. Spaces between these 2 were greater than normal and frequently filled with basement membrane-like material. (Keep this in mind for later when glycosylation is brought up). Permeability, meaning the ability to move water and chemicals through its walls) of diabetic blood vessels is present and may be explained by the spaces between the cells. These spaces may also explain retinopathy with anyeurisms (ballooning of vessel walls). Ballooning degeneration involving endothelial cells of cutaneous capillaries while leaving adjacent endothelial cells intact, was seen in 6 diabetic patients with early lesions of necrosis lipoidicum induced by trauma (Heng, Allen, Song, and Heng). Noted proliferation of endothelial cells obliterating vessel lumina may explain the paucity of dermal blood vessels in older lesions.

Membranocystic lesions, according to Sueki, were frequently found in skin diseases explained by diabetic microangiopathy (capillary disease). A person with blisters and 3 with front-of-the-leg patches had them. They occurred more often in diabetics with major complications - retinopathy, neuropathy, nephropathy. Other authors report ballooning of the blood vessel walls. Still others (Sueki et al.) describe structures of membranocystic lesions seen with the electron microscope. Tortuous thick bands composed of well-developed minute tubular structures, shrubbery-like structures made up of tiny cysts and microprojections, and thin membranes without minute tubular structures are observed. These may all derive from fat cells below the skin which become displaced into the skin so that they may be disposed of by appropriate cells.

Dr. Heinrich Koebner, in 1877, produced a typical psoriatic lesion in the unaffected skin of a psoriatic patient by inflicting trauma.

Since then, several skin diseases have been noted to appear after trauma. If pressure is accepted as a trauma, foot ulcers - certainly a skin condition - can, in part, be accounted for. Foot problems and amputations are so important in diabetic life that they deserve an article of their own, yet, they must at least be mentioned here. Callus is not more prevalent on diabetic feet than on normal feet but hemorrhage within plantar (sole) callus caused by diabetes was described. Hemorrhages were more prevalent in Type I than in Type II diabetics. Calluses certainly cause pressure and in a foot which has lost sensation, generate a focal point because the foot doesn't shift to spread the impact of weight-bearing. Callus may also act as a foreign body. Result: a hemorrhage or ulcer. It is also true that constant pressure on one spot can cause a callus. Foot ulcers in 54 diabetics were examined by Jones et al.. Abnormal pressure was judged to contribute to the formation of all ulcers associated with callus and definable trauma precipitated ulcer formation in 60% of all others.

Here is a quote from an abstract by Birrer and Rausher. I think it gives a good understanding.

A knowledge of anatomy, coupled with an awareness of biomechanical factors such as shoes, hosiery, and other environmental agents, provides sufficient expertise for treating the majority of foot ailments.

In 1984 Balkin suggested implanting fluid silicon beneath the skin to cushion pressure. The idea is intriguing but couple the fact that approval has not been granted by the FDA with the furor over leaking silicon from breast implants and it is probably best to leave the suggestion alone.

Agreement exists that wound healing is slow in diabetics but there is a lack of agreement on their predisposition to infections. Some think they suffer more infections. Other do not. When infections do occur they are hard to get rid of due to poor circulation and poor local nutrition. What does that mean?, you say. Poor circulation stops a good supply of oxygen, glucose (to be converted into energy), and medication from getting to the infected site. Killing power of diabetic's white blood cells is decreased by the lack of oxygen and high blood sugar levels. Erysipelas, defined as a febrile skin condition with sudden onset of a red, hard, expanding plaque with distinct border, has alcoholism, diabetes, and venous insufficiency as predisposing factors. In 52% of the cases Erysipelas originated from an infected ulcer. Streptococcus was frequently isolated (46%). Staphylococcus aureus (a very bad - difficult to treat bacterium) occurred in 59% of the cases and in 3 of these 122 cases it began growing in the blood stream (septicemia). Truly something to worry about. The patients were not all diabetics.

Previously undiagnosed Type IIs attended an Oral Medical Unit and upon the findings soon to be described, were tested and diagnosed. Of the 43 patients, 10 had prolonged fungal or bacterial infections and 6 had erosive mucosal lesions such as erosive lichen planus. Lichens are plants composed of algae and fungi living together happily. Fungi can lead the good life alone, too. Corneas obtained from the Medical Examiner's lab in Maryland were examined for pathogenic fungi. Comparing diabetic corneas with nondiabetic ones, 54% of the former cultured yeast while 35% of the later did. These could have been either normal fungal flora (all sorts of living things exist quite comfortably on our skin) or opportunistic fungal pathogens.

When toe-webs and toe-nails of still breathing diabetics were examined, 70 of the 73 (out of 100 diabetic participants) with clinical symptoms, revealed fungal elements. Clinical signs were present in 66 of 100 normal patients (isn't that an oxymoron?) but only 53 displayed fungal involvement. Interestingly, 100% of the patients with fungal infection had blood sugars of over 300 mg/dl (authors Alteras and Saryt). Diabetic women know this to be true because their vaginal Candida problems are much easier to control when blood sugars are down to a normal range (80-120 mg/dl). Yes, it's been confirmed by scientists. High blood sugars can be caused by infections (producing a vicious cycle of hyperglycemia caused by and encouraging infections). Hyperglycemia can lead to ketoacidosis and indeed, Tesfaye's group records 3 cases in which the causative infection was genital herpes. Their suggestion: examine patients in ketoacidosis for genital herpes. Another weird set of circumstances occurs when the patient presenting with hyperglycemic ketoacidosis is from sub-Saharan Africa. Guinea worms enter the sole of the foot with subsequent lichen infection. Early recognition and treatment brings a good outcome.

Hyperglycemia's most damaging effect may be the increase in nonenzymatic glycosylation it causes. What is that? Well, in a nonreversible chemical reaction, a molecule of glucose attaches to a molecule of protein. After that, these glycosylated proteins form crosslinks which then comprise large clumps of protein. Mechanically, such masses can interfere with things such as making the conduits in small blood vessels smaller still. The more glucose present, the more glycosylated proteins form. So diabetics with poor blood sugar control have more. (That is why glycosylated hemoglobin - HbA -measures past glycemic control. HbA disappears after 6-8 weeks because the red blood cells which contain it finish their lifecycles and are destroyed.) All right, hemoglobin is a protein that gets glycosylated but so is collagen, an important part of skin. Diabetics have thicker skin than normals and glycosylation of collagen may account for it.

According to Huntley, the yellowing of skin and nails, which is common among diabetic patients, may be due to the same process. In another paper this author states that diabetic thick skin of the extremities is apparently independent of the thickening skin processes associated with skin diseases. Examining diabetic thick skin microscopically, Hanna et al. described the collagen bundles as large, disorganized, and separated by clear spaces. Greater magnification showed thickened basement membrane (the membranes in cell walls) and extensive collagen polymerization - strands of the protein stuck together. An important experiment was performed by Sueki's group in which they took corneal and nail samples from non-diabetics and incubated them with glucose to cause glycosylation. Both tissues turned brown. Degree of browning increased with increasing quantities of glucose and with temperature. Conclusion: yellowing of skin and nails in diabetics may be due to glycosylation. This inference was confirmation of work done by Cerami and co-workers 10 years earlier.

Most proteins in living systems turn over with sufficient rapidity to avoid nonenzymatic browning but some, such as lens crystallins (accounting for diabetic cataract formation) and skin collagen, are exceptionally long-lived and may be vulnerable. The same process occurs in stored foods. Other cross-linkages of collagen also exist. Cross-linkages are present in all of us and may, in part, account for the aging process. Diabetics are said to age faster and perhaps the reason is that they have more glycosylated proteins. Related to this is the limited joint mobility which appears in some young diabetics.

Combine limited joint motion with thickened skin on the fingers and shortened extending finger muscles (present in many diabetics) and you come up with a condition in which the palms of the hands cannot flatten against each other. Think then. I have given you a picture of many colored diabetics who cannot physically pray. Not a pretty image. Fortunately most of us sugar-diseased people don't fit the portrait.

Usually it's just dry skin. Like many other aspects of diabetes, dry skin is a profit-making opportunity. In reading through a recent issue of a diabetes magazine published for patients, I noted 6 ads for dry skin products for diabetics - some for heels, some for fingers, some for general skin. Internationally, it's also money making. My daughter, who lives in Israel, recently brought me a gift of Dead Sea moisturizing lotion. She sees me so frequently rubbing in skin balms. However, I will have to ask her to explain to me why the logo on the bottle is of an ancient Egyptian woman.

Before the Diabetes Control and Complications Trial was reported, before angiotensin converting enzyme (ACE) inhibiting drugs were shown to slow the course of diabetic nephropathy, Barry, in 1991, wrote: "If we can prove that good blood glucose control and good blood pressure control can keep these terrible life complicating infirmities from happening, perhaps we can put greater stress on handling diabetes with a life style that will attain such conditions." Trying to guess what will happen tomorrow is hazardous unless you are privy to still restricted information that will influence the future. Barry had no such sources but in the quest to keep her readers advised took the plunge.

Predictions

"To predict", according to The Living Webster Encyclopedic Dictionary of the English Language, is to foretell, to prophesy. What has predicting to do with diabetes? Think. Prediction might allow interference, interference and possibly prevention of the disease and/or its complications. If we can identify those people who will get diabetes, we may be able to disrupt the march toward full blown illness.

It would seem that the development of diabetes is linked to the genetic makeup of the individual. IDDM (Type I or Insulin Dependent Diabetes Mellitus), according to recent studies, either is or isn't inherited, sometimes it seems to be and sometimes it just appears, but the likelihood of becoming diabetic is connected to the presence of certain specific genes. Which genes these are differs in different groups of humans. Among Caucasians the presence of genetic markers HLA 3 (Human Leukocyte Antigen), HLA 4, HLA 3/4, or DQ beta may indicate those who will develop diabetes. NIDDM (Type II or Non-Insulin Dependent Diabetes Mellitus) is more clearly inherited than IDDM but its genetic markers remain unknown.

If inheritance was the only cause for diabetes both twins in an identical pair would have the disease but this is not true in IDDM where only 25-50% of the pairs both are diabetic. However, if one twin has NIDDM in almost 100% of the cases the other identical twin will have it as well. The fact that twins are not equally afflicted by

IDDM strongly suggests the importance of the environment (prenatal, perinatal, or postnatal) in development of this disease. The story in NIDDM twins makes the identification of the responsible gene or genes an important piece of research. Nowadays, as gene manipulation becomes more possible and increasingly current, there is hope that we may be able to eliminate Type II diabetes. A complicating factor in understanding the genetics of diabetes is the early onset of IDDM which allows us to know the medical history of several generations of relatives but the late occurrence of NIDDM which does not.

One of the most exciting contemporary projects in medicine is human gene mapping. The goal of the so called genome project is to identify and know the link between each gene and what it controls. When this is finished, the gene or genes which cause diabetes will be identified and the people with this genetic defect can be treated before the symptoms of the disease appear. The genes themselves can be changed. Manipulation of genes lies in the not too distant future. Various groups of people show their diabetes in different ways (age of onset, fatness or thinness, inclination toward dehydration and ketoacidosis) and the causative genes may not be the same. It is not a simple problem. An ability to identify the genes which result in diabetes will be the ultimate predictor. At the stage we are now, knowing gene types in certain people allows us to foretell the possibility of diabetes and use other diagnostic tools to narrow the prophesy.

Foretelling Type I diabetes can be helped by determining the presence or absence of certain antibodies. As an autoimmune disease, diabetes can be thought of as rejection by the body of part of itself. In self rejection, individuals develops antibodies to themselves. We can identify 3 kinds of antibodies in diabetic persons. There are islet cell antibodies. When first degree relatives of diabetic children were examined for islet cell antibodies 3.1% had them. Riley et al showed that screening a large group (4015) of relatives detected 125 people with islet cell antibodies. IDDM developed in 40 of the 4015 and 27 of those 40 were islet cell antibody positive (67.5%). Another study identified children who were antibody positive and followed them for 6 years. Some of these children became negative. A small number (0.25%) of the islet cell antibody positive children developed IDDM so Karjalainen concluded that significant numbers were exposed to beta cell damage without progressing to IDDM. No child without islet cell antibodies became diabetic so the negative predictive value of the test was 100%.

While antibodies to insulin also exist and may have a prophesying role, the more exciting antibody (named for its weight), is called 64K. It can be present for as long as 7 years before the appearance of symptoms and shows up in 80% of those who will develop IDDM. Unfortunately 64K is very expensive to test for but now that it has been identified as glutamic acid decarboxylase, attempts can be made to clone it. After that, the test for 64K might possibly be produced via recombinant protein methods which would sharply reduce the cost. If testing were cheap, we might be able to survey the entire population and treat those who had the 64K antibody. Even if it remains an expensive procedure, and we devise methods to stop the development of diabetes, 64K testing may be less costly than a lifetime of diabetes which calls for a great outlay of money.

Immunosuppressive drugs given to individuals expressing diabetes related antibodies before the appearance of symptoms seem to prevent conversion to clinical diabetes for as long as the drugs are given. If immunosuppressive drugs such as cyclosporine are taken soon after the appearance of hyperglycemia there may be a return to normal blood glucose levels. The question that comes up is "Are the side effects of these drugs as devastating as the disease?". Another round of prediction would help. If we could know which diabetics would suffer complications (about 40% develop renal injury) we would know which ones to present with the idea of immunosuppressive drugs. Genetic determination of which diabetics will have to live with complications has been hinted at.

Not all diabetics suffer the terrible complications - the renal failure, vision loss, neuropathic manifestations. If we could foretell who would be afflicted and treat them with immunosuppressive drugs the remaining subjects could be allowed to just become diabetic.

It is the complications which make diabetes so costly (hospitalizations, doctors, medications, loss of work time) and so difficult to live with (foot problems, hypoglycemia, hyperglycemia, loss of vision, kidney failure, heart attacks, strokes, and so on). Or, if we can prove that good blood glucose control and good blood pressure control can keep these terrible life complicating infirmities from happening, perhaps we can put greater stress on handling diabetes with a life style that will attain such conditions. Of course it would be helpful if we could predict which people would comply with medical advice and which would not.

Finally, we can wish for an unclouded crystal ball or more scientific research to supply us with accurate looks into the future.

Starting at square 1, Barry in this 1991 column describes what happens to blood sugar levels in diabetes. Surprisingly, many otherwise sophisticated individuals with diabetes do not understand the basic abnormalities that accompany their disease. Typically straightforward writing communicates much in few words. Especially poignant is the passage on trying not to do away with yourself while juggling food and insulin.

Sugar - too much, too little

Diabetes mellitus was and is referred to as "the sugar disease". Too much sugar (hyperglycemia) occurs naturally in the blood stream and some tissues of diabetics. Too little sugar (hypoglycemia) usually results from doctor prescribed medications. Insulin or oral hypoglycemic agents are capable of lowering blood glucose levels to the point where distress develops. Both low blood sugar and high blood sugar spell trouble. Hypo- and hyperglycemia are life threatening circumstances making correct regulation of blood sugar the aim of all treatment.

Recognition of either state should not be a problem nowadays because rapid and inexpensive measurement of blood glucose levels is possible. In hospital emergency rooms, when comatose or "out of it" patients, or the elderly, or known diabetics arrive, blood sugar values should be determined. Simple, fast measurements are possible with finger stick, strip, meter technology.

Hyperglycemia accounts for approximately 1 in 1000 hospital admissions and 9% of all hospital admissions of diabetics. Aside from the very young, the majority of cases involve known Type I (Type I or Insulin Dependent Diabetes Mellitus) or undiagnosed Type II (Type II or Non-Insulin Dependent Diabetes Mellitus) diabetics. Previously diagnosed insulin-dependent diabetics who are seen in hyperglycemia usually have a history of multiple episodes of the same thing. Note that they should probably be better educated as to the causes of the condition and given hints as to how to avoid it.

A history of hyperglycemic episodes predisposes Type I diabetics to repetitions of the disorder for several reasons. While not the most important, mental causes are disturbing. Interruption of insulin delivery due to forgetting a dose or giving the wrong amount can be due to carelessness, incompetence or consciousness action (an attempt at passive suicide). Pancreatic Islet of Langerhans beta cell failure or insulin resistance can play parts. Mechanically, a clogged delivery system or an empty chamber in an insulin pump can account for insufficient insulin as can inaccurate syringe filling due to impaired vision. People can be too poor to afford the drug or live too far away from a convenient supply. Solutions exist but may not occur to those involved.

An overabundant secretion of counterregulatory hormones also explains high levels of glucose in the blood. Normal bodies not only produce insulin to keep blood sugar levels down but other hormones - glucagon, epinephrine, cortisol, and growth hormone - to raise blood sugar when it has fallen too low. After several years of living with their disease, diabetics (Type Is have already lost the ability to produce insulin) may no longer secrete sufficient amounts of glucagon and as the years go by many no longer manufacture enough epinephrine. Thus, the endocrine system which has balancing mechanisms built in, fails. The sugar rises. Stress can call upon the body to release these hyperglycemic-causing hormones.

Now we must examine the kinds of high blood glucose states that are seen. There is a condition called Diabetic Ketoacidosis (DKA) characterized by blood sugars of 300-350 mg/dl or higher (diabetics try to maintain at 80-140 mg/dl) and blood pH of less than 7.2 (normal blood pH is 7.4, a lower level indicates acidosis). As could be expected, there are patients with higher glucose levels who show no symptoms of DKA and those with lower values who do. Ketoacidosis refers to the acidity of the blood (pH less than 7.2) due to the presence of ketone bodies and ketone acids which, when in sufficient quantities, lead to a loss of bicarbonate and other body buffers. Remember back to high school science. Buffers help balance acids and bases and preserve the pH. Substantial deficits in sodium, potassium, magnesium, phosphorus, and water follow. Potassium shifts are most important but more about that later.

Glucose formation and ketone formation occur in the liver; when one increases the other does too. The presence of ketones and glucose in an acid urine confirms the diagnosis of DKA. Illness is held accountable for 50-60% of all DKA episodes. Emotional stress may also be very important but it has been poorly studied and is complicated. Think. Stress to one person may not be stress to another. In approximately 20-30% of DKA cases no precipitating circumstances can be found.

Absence or low levels of insulin are not always present in DKA. Indeed, the quantity of insulin may be normal but there is not enough to deal with the amount of glucose in the blood.

DKA deaths are greatest in the group of patients who are 65 years and older (around 10%) and are due in large part to coexistent illness. However, when coma and hypothermia are present, the death rate rises to 44%.

Mortality is higher (12-42%) in a second type of hyperglycemia called Hyperglycemic Hyperosmolar Coma (HHC). From the name you can suspect that patients are found in coma. HHC occurs in the very old and the very young, and most often in Type II diabetics while DKA is most common in Type I diabetics. Old age and social isolation predispose people to HHC. HHC happens more insidiously than DKA, so patients seek treatment later in the course of illness and when they are sicker. Here blood sugar levels are greater than 600 mg/dl and may rise to 2000 mg/dl, hyperosmolarity exists but significant ketoacidosis does not. Precipitating factors may include silent heart attacks (a complication of diabetes), pancreatitis, sepsis, stroke, or an array of drugs. In some individuals coma due to HHC may be the first evidence of diabetes.

No matter what the causative circumstances are, or how the hyperglycemic status is expressed - that is as DKA or HHC - dehydration results and is a major factor. Water loss can be through rapid acidotic breathing and the constant urination which is a symptom of uncontrolled diabetes. With lower fluid volume the kidneys filter less and so the proportion of glucose in the blood rises as does the proportion of ketone bodies. Dehydration may cause the release of counterregulatory hormones even though the level of sugar may not require them. Treatment of hyperglycemia is immediately concerned with correctly rehydrating patients. Since the dehydration is also intracellular, gently rehydrating brain cells before damage occurs is a great concern.

Plasma potassium concentration was mentioned before as being of critical importance. In DKA, the hydrogen ion shifts from the extracellular compartment to the intracellular compartment and the potassium ion goes the other way. Both an increase in the glucagon level and a decrease in the insulin level stimulate release of potassium from liver. Result - higher levels of potassium in the blood which is referred to as hyperkalemia. High potassium levels can lead to cardiac arrest - death.

In order to avoid the ultimate complication, treatment is started immediately and involves treating the dehydration and hyperglycemia. Volume replacement decisions include choice of correct fluid, amount, and rate of administration. Too great a degree of rehydration can cause pulmonary edema and congestive heart failure. Increasing blood volume automatically lowers the concentration of whatever is present in the blood. Glucose, potassium, and ketone concentrations are all shifted. Hyposmolar fluids should be used and the process must be done slowly.

At the same time, to treat DKA or HHC, insulin is administered to lower the blood sugar level. Years ago, large quantities, sometimes hundreds of units, were administered but now relatively small doses (5-6 units per hour) are given either IV or intramuscularly. In the hyperglycemic patient, insulin resistance has increased. Lowering sugar levels reverses this. The effect of treating with low amounts of insulin and not rapid fluid replacement is to avoid going too far and causing hypoglycemia and hypokalemia.

Constant monitoring of many things - glucose level, fluid level, potassium level and ECG tracings, to name a few - makes the process a busy, tiring time for the doctor but if it is not done correctly the complications which may occur, will require even more hours.

Suppose the hyperglycemia happens in a patient on dialysis where loss of water by urination cannot take place. Tzamaloukas and Avasthi of Albuquerque reporting in the Journal of Diabetic Complications worked with 23 episodes of hyperglycemia occurring in IDDMs on hemodialysis and 65 IDDMs on continuous peritoneal dialysis. High sugar in these patients is characterized by infrequent development of metabolic acidosis, frequent respiratory alkalosis, respiratory acidosis corrected by insulin therapy, and by metabolic alkalosis which develops during treatment. Administration of insulin corrects all the abnormalities though some more slowly than others. There were no differences noted between the two groups on two dialysis modalities. Another paper written by the same authors, however, indicates a dissimilarity. Here they state that the hemodialysis patient has a small shift in sodium content which they correct by drinking while the peritoneal dialysis patient who is losing fluid into the dialysate can achieve only partial correction through drinking. It all makes sense.

Loss of water seems to account for much of the disastrous circumstances associated with hyperglycemia. Preserving the amount of fluid in the body avoids many of the imbalances making the state of hyperglycemia less immediately threatening and easier to treat in the dialysis patient.

What then are our recommendations? Certainly not: All diabetics get thee to dialysis procedures. More justifiably - monitor your sugar levels. Keep yourself under reasonable control. And probably to all physicians - check everybody's blood glucose level and try to identify unknown diabetics.

Most known diabetics - surely the insulin taking variety - have experienced the other end of the blood sugar spectrum. Hypoglycemia happens about once a week in people taking two daily injections of insulin and may occur more frequently with more intensive therapy. As diabetic duration lengthens, the risk of low blood sugar incidents becomes larger because the dose of insulin required also becomes larger, glucagon release may be impaired, epinephrine release may be impaired, warning symptoms decrease, and because patients are human - those who have been free of insulin reactions take chances. Other causes contribute as well. Onset of menses, use of a new bottle of insulin, delayed stomach emptying, or a change of injection site may play a part. On the more depressing side overdoses of insulin can be used to commit murder or suicide.

In an attempt to not do away with themselves, diabetics daily play the game of balancing insulin dose, food intake, and exercise. Even without insulin, extreme malnutrition can cause low blood sugar as proved by a group of Jewish physicians in the Warsaw ghetto in 1941-42. Chronically malnourished or acutely food deprived people who consume moderate to large amounts of alcohol can experience hypoglycemia in 6-36 hours. Such "drunks" may be found the next morning, dead in the jail cell where they were placed to sober up.

Not at all the person's fault are the insulin producing tumors which occasionally grow. They make blood sugar control very difficult.

Fortunately, the signs and symptoms of low blood sugar usually follow the same pattern in a given individual although what they are changes over the years. With a mild insulin reaction, adrenergic symptoms (tachycardia, palpitations, shakiness) or cholinergic symptoms (sweating) or nervous system symptoms (inability to concentrate, dizziness, hunger, or blurred vision) are felt. Giving yourself a simple carbohydrate - sugar in any form - takes care of the problem. Learn to always have something within easy grasp. In a severe reaction, help must be given by another person. For this reason it is important that people around you know that you are diabetic and understand what to do for you. Of most concern are the diabetics who experience no signs of hypoglycemia for various reasons.

The key to avoiding most low sugar incidents is education. Learning to recognize what is happening to you, how to predict the possibility and correct it either through adjusting food intake or drug dose should help. It won't eliminate all episodes but should make them fewer.

Both hypo and hyperglycemia tend to recur in individuals so take that as an excuse to be extra careful. Even diabetics are significant to the rest of the world.

The downside of improved metabolic regulation of blood glucose — repetitive episodes of hypoglycemia (low blood sugar) can be terrifying causing loss of intellectual competence and even coma. Barry speculates in this 1993 column that the cumulative penalty for avoidance of eye and kidney complications by tight glucose control just might be a reduction in brain mass and the ability to reason. Yet another reason to hope for alternative approaches to diabetic management.

I'M *TRYING* TO THINK !

Let me quote from Ellenberg and Rifkin's Diabetes Mellitus: Theory and Practice Fourth edition. "Hypoglycemia is a fact of life for people with insulin dependent diabetes mellitus." Glucose is an obligate metabolic fuel for the central nervous system... Thus survival of the brain—and therefore the individual—is dependent upon a continuous supply of glucose. Even brief hypoglycemia can cause profound dysfunction of the brain; prolonged severe hypoglycemia can cause brain death."

That says it all. The brain burns only sugar and when it is low on sugar it doesn't work right. Perhaps I should leave the rest of this article blank. But I won't.

My concern today is the effects of hypoglycemia — low blood sugar — on the brain. Depending on which measuring system you use, low blood sugar is defined as a level below 55 mg/dl or 3 mmol/L. (That may be the scientific definition but I am in trouble when my sugar is 70mg/dl or lower.) Whether some or all of the consequences of hypoglycemia happen right then and there, or have a long term effect, must be explored.

What do we mean by effects on the brain? What is brain function? Is there really a difference in the working of the brain between chemically caused and psychologically caused mental disease? For my purposes, I think not. Even if you are a devotee of psychological causes for mental illness, you must concede that brain cells are involved in the process, and therefore, the chemical state of the cells is important. Sugar is the only thing the brain can burn to get its energy. Low fuel— low function.

The brain controls total body. Responsible for motion, sensation and thought, the brain is affected in all these areas by insufficient energy. For the most part, I will discuss only "thought" function.

Hypoglycemia can cause a range of symptoms from subtle cognitive impairment to seizures, and even loss of consciousness.

Fatigue, dizziness, visual changes, abnormal sensations such as prickling or tingling - particularly around the mouth - and hunger, can occur. Insulin taking diabetics, when their blood sugar is low, can act like they are drunk (a good reason to wear medical identification), show poor judgement, act or move in repetitive patterns, or just plain be uncooperative. As a little side trip, let me tell you some of my experiences.

When I first became an IDDM (Insulin Dependent Diabetes Mellitus or Type I diabetic) and my sugar went down, my brain would tell me: "First finish what you are doing and then get sugar." Trouble. Trouble. It was necessary to put much effort into fighting this. GO. TAKE CARE OF YOURSELF AND THEN COME BACK. It's taken years, but now I can laugh when I react that way and handle the situation correctly. More recently my problem is sight. After cleaning my glasses for the seventh time, I silently shout at myself: IDIOT. IT'S NOT YOUR GLASSES. YOU'RE LOW SUGAR. I do wonder what my next difficulty will be. I know I'm not thinking right when I'm having an insulin reaction. I can't read. I can't concentrate. And I'm not physically well coordinated either. By the way, how many of you get overpoweringly sleepy like me, when the sugar level rises?

Funny situation. Diabetic wife gets argumentative when her glucose level falls. Every time she starts to quarrel, husband grabs food and feeds her. She complains — one of the great pleasures of married life, *FIGHTING*, is now denied her.

There seems to be no argument that insulin reactions cause thinking problems. A question came up as to whether low blood sugar levels in nondiabetics would cause the same thing. Work, published in 1993 by Mitrakou et. al,, showed lowering the sugar levels in 10 normal volunteers, caused no change in cognitive function when the sugar level was lowered rapidly over a period of 30 minutes. However, when the sugar was lowered in a stepwise manner, cognitive function did deteriorate at the lowest plateau which was 42 mg/dl (2.3 mmol/L). It is my contention that diabetes changes the body in many ways. Perhaps this experiment does not account for the behavior of a diabetic body which is different from a normal body, possibly explaining why diabetics have problems *no matter which way* the sugar is lowered.

A study done by the Lingenelser group in 1992, used 10 IDDMs. They found a significant reduction in thought processes in 8 of the patients during hypoglycemia. A level of 39 mg/dl was used as the hypoglycemic state. Motor task performance also got worse and the patients feelings of well being deteriorated.

1993 brought the idea that the 2 halves of the brain might be affected differently by low blood sugar. Right and left hemispheres seem to control various functions so perhaps they have unlike reactions to low glucose. Nope.

Maybe the level of glucose necessary for people to have hypoglycemic symptoms varies and indeed, it seems to. Levels necessary to cause cognitive dysfunction are not the same in all of us.

Other things to think about include musing over the effect of age of onset and therefore age of hypoglycemic episodes, on brain function. Early age of onset and frequency of low blood sugar events were found, by Bischoff, Warzak, Maguire, and Corley, to be highly related to significant defects in intellectual and academic performance.

Is there an effect on schoolwork for students? Are they perhaps, less intellectual than they would be if they hadn't become diabetic at a very early age? Does that matter since they *are diabetic?* According to the Ellenberg/Rifkin, text onset of diabetes before the age of 5 produces some cognitive deficit. The thought is that hypoglycemia before the central nervous system has fully matured may be the cause and that severe hypoglycemia may yield irreversible neurological disturbances. Kids with on-again/off-again low blood sugars during the school day may show poor school performance.

If the reason or mechanism for intellectual impairment due to low blood sugar is discovered perhaps it can be interfered with. Richardson tells us that postmortem studies suggest central nervous system degeneration (and that includes the brain) in people who had diabetes mellitus. The cognitive deficits shown by Type I diabetics tend to be relatively minor and independent of clinical symptoms. It is also true that different studies report different deficiencies; Richardson claims that this inconsistency is typical of nervous system pathology. Type II diabetics show a more consistent pattern of what is wrong — their problems include learning and memory — and correlate with the blood glucose level. On an upbeat note the researcher says all of this is unlikely to interfere significantly with patients' everyday functioning. OK I'll go along with that *except if the patient is a student or involved in making on-the-spot decisions.*

In order to judge long term after effects of hypoglycemia on adult Type I diabetics, 2 groups were tested. One consisted of 10 non-diabetic people and a group of 55 insulin dependent diabetics matched not only in age but in more psychological aspects such as professional and social status. A set of 30 diabetics who had suffered frequent severe attacks of hypoglycemia and were unaware of the onset of hypoglycemia, was compared with a set of 25 patients who were aware of hypoglycemia. Both groups had had diabetes for approximately the same length of time, had approximately the same range of glucose control, and showed similar degenerative complications. All patients were tested when they were not hypoglycemic. Normals showed the best scores. Diabetics who were aware of low sugar when it occurred, scored significantly better than diabetics who were unaware of their low sugar levels. The authors conclude that severe hypoglycemia may have a deleterious effect on cognitive performance and that several severe episodes could be responsible for permanent mental impairment. Keep this in your mind. I will bring it up again during my summing up.

Ryan, Williams, Feingold and Orchard came up with the same results but they emphasized the presence of neuropathy rather than the presence of hypoglycemic unawareness to explain the correlation. A possibility that hypoglycemic unawareness is due to neuropathy presents itself. Do other causes exist? The body responds to low levels of glucose in the blood by releasing hormones, called counter regulatory hormones, whose actions cause the production of glucose from storage in the liver and muscles and its discharge into the blood thus raising its level. Indeed, normal blood sugar levels are maintained by a balance of insulin, which lowers the level, and the other hormones, which raise it. Counter regulatory hormones may have as one of their physiological actions, perception of low blood sugar. In general, the longer the course of diabetes, the poorer the body responds with these hormones thus battling low blood sugar less well. I find myself wondering if there is a difference in the level of circulating counter regulatory hormones between diabetics who experience frequent insulin reactions and those who have them infrequently.

Deeper understanding of the effects of hypoglycemia were looked into by a team led by Bendtson. Morning cognitive function tests were done on 8 Type I diabetics. The experiment was set up in an interesting way. Each patient acted as both experimental subject and control. During control nights blood sugar of at least 5 mmol/L was maintained. During experimental nights glucose levels were dropped to less than 3 mmol/L. No difference in testing showed up but there were disturbances in sleep patterns. With hypoglycemia, the amount of deep sleep was reduced. Remember my comment about getting very sleepy when my sugar level is rising after an insulin reaction? Maybe there is a connection.

In 1992, the Blackman group worked with poorly controlled IDDMs. Their cognitive function when their sugar was near normal was the same as that of nondiabetics but they did show a longer time necessary to react to visual stimuli. During low blood sugar both cognitive function and reaction time to seeing something, deteriorated. As sugar levels were raised both of the measured functions returned to normal but more slowly than in the normal control subjects.

According to a team led by Deary, frequent severe hypoglycemic episodes slightly lowered the performance and verbal IQ but when number of incidents was controlled, differences in performance IQ disappeared. Significant correlation between the frequency of insulin reactions and magnitude of intellectual decline was reported by Langan et al.

Be aware that there are studies which detect no cognitive function dysfunction due to hypoglycemia. Whether or not there are effects on the brain of low blood sugar is thus, a gray, not black and white, area.

Going back to the question of psychological aftermaths on the insulin taking diabetic mind, note that there is no such thing as a "diabetic personality". Not clear too, is the amount of mental disorders present among diabetics. Is it equal to, less than, or more than among nondiabetics? Not known. However, consider the impact of hypoglycemia on sex life, social relations, depression, and anxiety disorders. Think of anorexia and bulimia. Think of the stress generated by attempts to control glucose level.

Hypoglycemia is important in terms of functioning. I am concerned by the recently reported DCCT (Diabetes Control and Complications Trial) which casually listed as a side effect of tight blood sugar control, a ***THREE FOLD*** increase in frequency of ***SEVERE*** hypoglycemic episodes. With the good there comes the bad. Insulin is a wonder. It saves lives but longer diabetic life leads to major complications in many patients. More normal blood glucose levels may slow or alleviate eye, kidney, and nerve complications in 70%, 50%, or 60% of patients but what will be the effect of frequent severe hypoglycemic episodes? Unknown. I worry about jumping out of the frying pan into the fire.

Here I go — off to eat a french fry!

Short Stories

Like actors, writers continuously seek employment while learning to endure rejection. Barry was indefatigable in pursuit of gaining publication for her work. Refusal after refusal did not stop yet another submission. Ultimately, success — meaning acceptance for cash — came though too infrequently. This story, based on a newspaper report of an event in a nearby Greek Diner, was sold to Greek Accent and published in their May 1987 issue (pp 33-35).

The Attacker and the Waitress

George looked up from his cash register and watched in disbelief as the bearded young man marched from the direction of the kitchen toward the diner's front door with a waitress slung over shoulder. As her boss, he knew the girl. Alice was an ordinary person, with an ordinary life—or so George had thought, when he thought of her at all.

Neither the stance of the restaurant owner's short, rotund figure nor the dark thickly lashed, flashing eyes set in the round face gave a clue to his reaction. Would he be chivalrous or think only of himself and his business? Should he worry about protecting the money in the drawer in front of him or the young woman who was punching, hitting and kicking the man who was carrying her? Whichever way George went, it would be total involvement.

Later, in the ambulance, still bleeding and in pain, he smiled. His father would have been proud of him for defending the weaker sex. And he had done that successfully. The girl was unhurt. She wasn't the kind of girl his father would have respected, but then morals had changed. All the young people seemed to live together these days and there was nothing unusual about her wanting to leave this particular lover. Breaking up a live-in arrangement was frequent. But she should have known he was a violent person. After all, she knew he was a cop. Now there are gentle cops and hard cops and all kinds of cops, but each seems to have a violent streak. There were no doubts in George'smind when he saw the man striding through the restaurant, first by himself and a few seconds later with his burden, that savagery was natural to him.

"Put her down! Put her down! Get out of my restaurant! Out! Ooof!" The punch to his belly hurt and sent George sprawling to the floor.

"Get out of my way. She is coming home with me!" the intruder shouted, with the waitress still thrown over his shoulder. "She's my girl!"

Fearful of the outcome of his action, George grabbed for the man's leg and brought him down. Enraged, the youth raised his fist.

"Don't hit me. Don't hurt me. Oh, Jesus!" half screamed, half groaned George, as punches and kicks landed on him. He felt the pain of the blow to his groin, heard the bone snap in his leg, realized he had broken a toe when his foot got caught in the rung of the chair that was swung at him, knew he was being punched in the kidneys, was sure his eye was turning black and blue after his head hit the edge of the table. Finally, feeling inadequate he gave up. He had landed only a few whacks on the body of the man who was beating him.

Through a blur, George knew that there were others in the brawl. He heard Spanish curses. Listened to the sounds of fist and feet meeting flesh. Was aware of someone calling the police. Saw out of half closed eyes, the girl standing to one side. Realized there was a crowd around them. Felt pain and fainted. Days after, lying in his hospital bed, when he was questioned by the detectives, he got as much information as he gave. The big burly one told him that Gary, "the perpetrator," had left the scene and was picked up later. One of the customers had been an off-duty cop who recognized Gary as a fellow officer and refused to arrest him. Both the cook and the busboy, Joe and Abel, who had joined in the fight were in the hospital—a different one. One of them was badly hurt. The other was soon to be released with a broken arm.

"I'll call them up this afternoon," thought George.

He gave the detectives as much as he could remember. They said they would be back and asked him to try to think of anything to add to his story.

After they left, he became worried about the diner. Who was running it? Was it open? How much damage had been done? How could he find out? His head throbbed. Clear thinking was difficult if not impossible. Mental exertion made him tired and he fell asleep only to be awakened an hour later by the ringing of the telephone.

"Hello, George?"

"Dimitri! How is the diner? How are you? What's happening? Who...?"

Laughing, Dimitri said, "Slow down. First things first. How are you feeling? I came to see you yesterday but you were so out of it you didn't know I was there. Better today? Can I come and see you soon?"

"Better. Better. Yes, come and visit. But now tell me about the business."

"Didn't know whether it would be what you wanted but I m running the place. Thomas opens up in the morning. I come in at around noon and stay up till closing time. The whole staff is being great. No arguments. No fusses. Wait till you get back. The fur will fly again. Right now though, they re trying to make it easy for me. We've cleaned up the breakage. Replaced the one smashed window and threw out the splintered table and crushed chairs. Makes for more space in the dining room. The insurance company wants to talk to you and have you file a claim. The breakage is covered and the medical expenses for all three of you. Those guys sure put up a fight, just like you did."

"Tell me. I don't remember it and it's driving me crazy, lying here bandaged and splinted and casted and not knowing what happened."

"Remember how it started? After you landed on the floor he kept kicking you in the head, in the back, between the legs. You grabbed for him and landed a few hits, but not much. Joe and Abel came running at the same time and piled into him. He fought like a tiger—got them both on the floor a couple of times. People were standing around watching. They moved back when the action got close to them but it took a little while before someone realized they should call the police. In the ten minutes before the prowl car came, the guy ran out leaving the girl there. Some other people left. Probably didn't want to get involved as witnesses. And this one fella, we've seen him come in uniform, he left too. An ambulance arrived a little later. Somebody called for another one, and they took you away first. The girl told them who the assailant was and where he lived. We shut the diner down for the rest of the night and cleaned up as best we could. Say, you'll need a lawyer. Do you know one? Can I call him for you? Want it to wait until I see you? You've got enough to think about now."

"I can't remember. What's her name? You know. The girl."

"Alice. Alice-what, I don't know. I can look it up in the payroll if you want."

"The police want me to press charges. I've got to think it out, to sort it out. Thanks for calling. See you when you get here. I think I'll just sleep now."

Who was this out-of-uniform cop who left? Why did he leave? What sort of guy was Gary? What did he do for a living? Oh yeah, he was a cop. Why had Alice left him? Questions, questions, questions. Maybe he would start getting answers soon.

There weren't many visitors. George had neither wife nor children. He had arrived in New York from his native Greece at the age of 25 and been busy ever since making a living. Trying to get himself established, social life was not on his schedule. Occasionally he thought of getting married and having kids. Fatherhood would be right up his alley. Patience and caring about the feelings of others were part of him. When, on occasion, a child reached for him and hugged, the feeling of happiness was marred by the realization of what was missing. A feeling of loneliness crept into his soul but never showed on his face; the smile remained. He seldom met a woman who attracted him, and when he did he was scared to find out whether she would pay him any attention.

Shyness didn't shine through in his other meetings with people. He enjoyed standing at the front of his restaurant, greeting customers, cordial to the newcomers, warm and friendly to the regulars. Some asked questions which he tried his best to answer. At times he even went to the kitchen to get lists of ingredients or suggestions from the cook, and once went so far as to drag a huge bag of pancake mix out to the dining room. Anything to please a customer. His middle was proof of the quality of his food. At Christmas time he needed no padding to play St. Nick.

Joe and Abel did come towards the end of his hospital stay. His room echoed the boiling of the melting pot that is New York. George's Greek accent mingled with Joe's Haitian tones and Abel's Columbian ones. After reminiscing about the fight and saying that they all were glad to still be alive, the visitors expressed their fear of getting involved in legal battles. Illegal alien status complicates life. They had to quit their jobs and disappear.

"How am I going to get other guys as good as you two? Go. Go. You have to protect yourselves first. I'll call Dimitri. Meet him at the diner and he'll have money for you to get you started. Good luck. Let me hear from you. And—thanks."

The next few months were busy, occupied with court appearances, stays, delays, a trial, newspaper interviews, appointments with the Assistant District Attorney who was involved because of the disappearing cop. Seems that he had recognized Gary as a fellow officer and had not wanted to interfere. Other professions protect their own—notoriously doctors and lawyers—but this case was different. Physical damage was involved.

After more than a year that man in blue was called up on charges by the Police Department. Loyalty to a fellow cop would have been praised under other circumstances. But all he was found guilty of was misjudgment. The fight had been over by the time he got to the scene. Sitting in the back of the restaurant the ruckus didn't come to his notice until he went up front to pay.

As the days passed and more and more customers saw the notice on the diner door asking for witnesses to step forward, and did, George's spirits rose. He still hurt. He wasn't healed yet, but the thought that people liked and respected him well enough to give their time and energy for his defense pleased him. When he thought of their response, warmth spread from his sewn up scalp to his broken little toe. That guy had really done a job on him.

It took six weeks after his release from the hospital before he was well enough to return to work. Most people who ate at the diner were aware of the story and George was greeted with interest and affection. The restaurant had been the center of his life since he opened it six years earlier, but now it was his whole focus. He vowed to update it, to serve bigger portions, to get better cooks, to make it more attractive. He spent longer hours there. Home was just a place he went to sleep.

"Hey George, I heard that guy who beat you up got out. How much time did he do? Four months? Doesn't seem enough for a guy who beat up three of you. But that's the system. What cha gonna do?"

George leafed through the pile the mailman had delivered. He smiled when he saw the restaurant journal he had been waiting for and immediately found the table of contents. Several articles caught his attention. Scanning them, he tried to think if he could use their information and ideas in his diner—the diner that was the whole center of his world. He loved keeping up with the trade and read all the magazines published about restaurants. Bills and junk mail made up the rest of the stack, except for one item. Puzzling over what it was, he slit the envelope open and found a wedding invitation. It was simple but in good taste. He was stumped by the names of the bride and groom. Looking at the envelope to make sure it was his mail, the address astonished him. "George, Atheneum Diner, 460 Prospect Ave., Brooklyn, N.Y. 11241." And then, the truth struck him. It was them—the attacker and the waitress.

Should he go? Should he send a gift? What was he supposed to do? What was he supposed to feel?

"They'll probably name their first baby after me!" That was the thought that flashed through his mind as he turned to the cash register to take the money a customer was handing him.

Written in 1987, this short story is one of Barry's first attempts at being a short story writer. It is as fresh today as it was when first conceived. Barry's letter of transmission to potential publishers stated: "Bibliographically, I'm not the usual model. Writing is my third career and I have medical columns in 3 kidney patient magazines. Starting as a bacteriologist, I graduated to teaching first grade, and then, with failing health, to sitting at home. Diabetes caused my eyes and kidneys to fail at the same time. Thanks to modern medicine, I have my sight back and thanks to a loving sister who donated a kidney I do fairly well in that department, too. The diabetes remains."

Forgive Me Jack. Love, Pop

He arrived at the meeting place early and waited for his son. It was fall. A lovely day was on its way yet the sun was not up at 7:00 in the morning. The colors of the leaves would appear soon, brilliant against a vivid blue sky. Few cars drove down Fifth Avenue and the noise of the occasional bus didn't quite blot out the roaring of the lions in the zoo. The amalgam of sights and sounds and smells were not what most people identified with the Big Apple but they were quintessential New York. African and metropolitan sounds mingled with New England foliage, here at the edge of Central Park, as they did nowhere else in the world. Rush hour brought street vendors selling breakfast foods. Odors from exotic places tantalized the nose, saliva filled the mouth and sensations of "empty" assailed the stomach. Dog spoor stench cut across pleasing aromas. None of it entered John's heightened awareness of the space around him. He was waiting for his son.

Standing in a doorway across the street from the fountain which tumbled and gurgled in front of the hotel, he watched two young men amble near the bubbling water, take a few steps this way and a few that way but not leave, staying close. As the minutes went by more just-out-of adolescence males appeared and strolled around the area. The square began to crowd.

John was filled with apprehension. Did he want his son to appear or didn't he? It had been a while since he had seen Jack. What had the boy been doing? Boy. Was he still a boy or had he become a man. Boy. Man. Man. Boy. Son. Nonson.

"You're not my son anymore. My son wouldn't have done that. Wouldn't have slapped his mother. Get out of my house. Get. . ."

"But Pop. She's drunk again."

"She tries. Didn't she cook supper last night?"

"Yeah. Last night. But it's only afternoon and she's been at the bottle so hard she doesn't know what's going on. Thought maybe I could bring some friends around. She opened the door in an old dirty house dress that wasn't even buttoned. Her hair's a mess. She stinks. She says dirty things. I got them outa there so fast. . ."

"You gotta respect her. Maybe if you'd come in first your friends wouldn't of barged in. They don't belong here anyway. Why'd you hit her?"

"I came home, like you did, wanting supper. She wasn't in the kitchen cooking. She wasn't even passed out quietly on the couch. She was in **my** room. Pulling out **my** things. Everything was all over. Clean clothes. Dirty clothes. Magazines. School papers. Marbles. Deodorant. What a mess. Why didn't you get her out of there? You're her old man."

"It's a sickness. You don't get mad at someone whose got TB or cancer."

"No. But you get them help when they need it and they don't pull your life apart. I can't bring anyone home. **I** can't come home. There's nothing here for me. You say you don't want me hanging around. Where am I supposed to go? Do your homework. Where? Eat good food. How am I supposed to get it? Don't skip breakfast. Half the time the only thing in the refrigerator is a couple of bottles of beer. I can't stand it anymore. I've got an address but no home."

"If it's so bad - leave."

"Even you couldn't stop her. I didn't want any more of my things thrown around. The only way I could stop her was to hit her. She stopped."

"You can't hit your mother. Get out of here. Take your things. Go. I don't want to see you anymore. You're not my son."

And so Jack left. Hoisting across his shoulder the duffel bag that held his things, he slammed the door and was gone. Five months had passed and there was no word from him. Not a telephone call. Nothing.

John felt empty. Maggie seemed drunk all the time. The house was a mess, dirty, empty of even simple food. If he didn't stop at the store and bring something home with him neither of them ate. He was tired of tuna fish, cheese sandwiches, canned macaroni and cheese, hot dogs and no companionship. Scolding, sympathy, shaking, refusing to give her money, nothing worked. Maggie got her booze and drank. All the chores of the household were on John's shoulders. He was weary of doing laundry, cleaning, making the bed, washing dishes and earning their money at his job. He'd never liked being a bus driver anyway. He often thought of joining her and sliding into degradation at her side. But - but - there was Jack. Or was there Jack? Where was Jack? Would he ever find him? What would he tell him if he found him? What could he do? Where would Maggie drag him? Exhausted by problems that seemed to have no solutions, he left Maggie sitting in the kitchen, staring into space and went to bed.

Over the weeks a plan formed in his mind. He would look up "alcoholic" in the phone book and find a place where he could commit Maggie. Or he would leave her. Years ago he had loved her when she was a pretty, alive and loving girl. He didn't think he would ever know what had changed her but he sure didn't love her now. He didn't think he owed her anything either. He'd tried. He'd made a home, earned money, enough money for them to live on, loved his son. The change in her was slow. At first there had been the smell of alcohol and later the sights of drunkenness. He'd thought that it would pass. It never had. She'd gotten fat, wrinkled. That wouldn't have bothered him if she'd kept the sweetness and cared for him or for their son. She had become the center and only occupant of her universe. Two of them were left outside in the cold. John and Jack hadn't drawn together but pulled at each other, argued and grew silent - until the night when Jack left.

I've got to find him. But how? I remember a story I saw on TV. This man wanted to get his girl back. He put an ad in the paper. What are they called? Oh yeah, personals. It's got to be worded just right. I want to tell him that I'm sorry. I want him for my son. I miss him. I'm worried about him. I have a plan for Ma. I won't let her hurt him anymore. I want him to come home. Sad and dejected he crawled into bed beside the already snoring Maggie.

Next day, on his way to work, he bought a newspaper. At lunch opening to the ads, he read the personals. Trying and trying he couldn't fit all his words into a good order to make them say what he wanted. Seeing how similar the ones in print were, he though **his** would have to jump off the page at the reader. He would have to make it different somehow. For the first time in months he felt happy, involved, hopeful. That night studying the page again, the little sidebar that suggested calling for help with writing an ad, caught his eye. Opening the container of ice cream he had brought home, he dished out some for Maggie and some for himself. She wasn't as far out of it as usual and ate a bit, even smiling as the cold sweet slid down her throat. To lighten his mood even further there were no horrible stories on the 10 o'clock news.

Next day he approached his supervisor. “Dick, I've gotta make an important phone call today. Is there some time when your office is empty and I could use it? All the years I've been working out of this garage and I've never asked a thing.”

"Use my desk. Use the phone. Take as long as you need. I'll go to lunch when you come in for your lunch break. Glad it's such an easy favor."

And so at 12:20, John knocked on the door. Waving at him, Dick left and John stood unsurely at the threshold. He wanted his son. One foot in front of the other he walked resolutely to the desk and sat down. From the plastic shopping bag he clutched in his hand he removed some blank paper, the sheet he had written his important points on, the newspaper page and two pencils (he'd learned in school to have two in case one broke). Pulling the phone to him, he stared at it for a long moment and then dialed.

"Advertising department, Miss Susy speaking."

"Uh. I want to place an ad but I've never done it before and I don't know how."

"What kind of an ad?"

"Umm. Personal."

"You want Miss Ruth. Hold on and I'll transfer you."

This was getting to be too much. Should he hang up? He was scared. What if the connection was broken? Simple obstacles to his plan loomed large. Tension made everything seem giant. Fortunately the telephone was answered by Miss Ruth quite quickly.

"How can I help you?"

Thank heavens. A friend.

"I want to place an ad, a personal ad, but I don't know how to make it sound right."

"I'll help. That's my job. Now let's start. Who is it for?"

"Jack. He's my son."

"What do you want it to say?"

"All is forgiven. I have a plan to end our problem. I want you to come home. Come and talk to me at least. We won't meet at the house but somewhere else. I guess maybe the fountain in the square at 59th and Fifth. If we make it early in the morning maybe we can spend the whole day together. Please meet me. I love you."

"That's an awful lot for a little ad. Let's see. "All is forgiven. Please meet me at the 59th St. and Fifth Avenue fountain at 8 A.M. on Thursday the 14th so we can talk over my plans. Love, Pop."' How does that sound?"

"It's good. It's good, but I want it to jump off the page so he'll notice it."

"Well we could do double or triple size with bigger print. That'll cost you more, of course."

"I don't care. I want him to see it. Is it in for only one day?"

"No. It runs for a full week and we'll start it a week before the 14th. All right?"

"I'll get a money order on my lunch break tomorrow. Who should I have it made out to?"

Hanging up the phone he shoved the papers back into his bag and left the office, closing the door behind him.

Occupied with buying the money order, mailing it off and then waiting for the 7th to arrive so he could see his ad, days flew by and life seemed pleasant.

There it was:

Jack,
All is forgiven. Please meet me at the
5th Ave. and 59th St. fountain at 8 A.M. on
Thursday the 14th so we can talk over my plans.
Love, Pop

While the week before had raced past this one dragged. John worried. Would Jack see the ad? Would he answer it? Did he want to be the son again?

Finally the day arrived and John got to the square at 7:00. No one was there. Afraid to stand right out in the open he went across the street and occupied a doorway. At 7:30, coming from different directions, two young men appeared and dawdled around the fountain. By 7:40 there were twenty and by 7:45 a crowd of 50 mingled in the space. At 8:00 several hundred men filled the zone.

John felt lost. He knew that if he called "Jack", voices from all the throats would answer. So many Jacks. So many problems. So much love waiting for a father.

Feeling despondent, John thought he would leave the growing crowd but he couldn't bring himself to just walk away. His eyes searched the faces, some young, some old, of the fellows milling about. Once he thought he caught sight of *his* Jack but it turned out to be a stranger. His feet shuffled across the plaza. The group thinned as he approached its edge. One figure stood out. Away from the group, back turned, shoulders drawn down in disappointment but it looked familiar to John. *Could it be?* Slowly he approached. The form bent a little, just enough to show the face. John cried out in delight and relief: "Oh Jack. Oh Jack. You came. You came." And the two of them hugged.

"Dad. Are you all right? How's Mom? I've missed you so. What solutions? What plans? Have you really come up with something to do? Can I come home? I'll help. It's been so lonely."

A few minutes later, sitting quietly over a cup of coffee, the future was discussed. Not everything was clear but one thing was for sure. It would be a future together.

Written in 1993, Barry in 1997 characterized this unpublished piece in a letter of transmission to a publisher: "Maiya's Daughter is a 3,300 word short story dealing with the major modern problem of child care. Maiya solves it in a unique manner which gets her into trouble. Unable to afford available baby sitting services and closed out by the long waiting lists for free assistance, she locks the girl and supplies in her car trunk. Reported to the police by a nosy neighbor, Maiya is accused of child abuse, is severed from her baby and jailed. Thanks to her boss's intervention the ending is upbeat."

Maiya's Daughter

Carrying the sleeping child from the car, Maiya looked around the third floor apartment glad it wasn't up two more flights, Tiredness surrounded her and she needed to sleep. Her thoughts were fuzzy. Bette, already in her pajamas, shifted slightly and then curled up comfortably, as her body tumbled into bed.

Maiya quickly stepped into the bathroom, stripped, took off her makeup, and climbed into the shower. No more than half an hour passed between the key in the door and the scramble into bed. She pulled the blanket up over Bette, cuddling her. Sleep came quickly.

If she could see herself she would note a small, plump, olive-skinned woman with short wavy dark hair. A woman who kept herself clean and dressed in simple clothes often made of patterned cloth. She would find herself watching a quiet, calm person who smiled easily and loved to laugh. But she couldn't see herself and wasn't much interested in her own looks anyway. The dark brown eyes remained closed until Bette woke her up in the morning.

Giggling, Bette shouted: "I'm hungry Mommy. Wake up. Wake up."

And, covering her ears, Maiya did.

"Good morning. Give me a kiss..........and a hug. Out you go. Potty!"

Soon the teakettle whistled with hot water for coffee. Oatmeal simmered. One wall held all the kitchen stuff. There were a small stove, matched in size by a small refrigerator, a sink, almost-not-worth-counting counter space and cupboards under and over everything. A 3x5 formica table and three wooden chairs sat a little off to the side. She had chosen to paint the one big room bright yellow and had poorly, but determinedly, stitched white curtains, with yellow flowers for both windows. A double bed covered by cheerful sheets and a plaid blanket took up one corner. Couch, TV on a stand and three lamps managed to fill the remaining area. Tub, toilet, sink left little space to turn around in the bathroom and the single closet felt equally confining.

But she could afford it - barely - and she never paid the rent late. Pride for that occupied a corner of her mind.

"Come up on the couch and watch your program", suggested Maiya.

With her child happily settled, she cleaned up from breakfast, made the bed and studied the contents of the refrigerator. Pretty empty. Today would be a shopping day. Enough eggs for two days' lunches, baked beans for another, tuna, soup, and the staples - bread and milk.

As she watched Bette totally involved in her TV program, Maiya mentally hugged herself. Was she doing right for the little girl she loved so much? Was it right to work to support them and not take welfare? How could she explain to somebody else how she managed child care? Nobody to talk about it with. No family. No friends. And certainly no husband. As a good woman, she tried to manage their lives the best way she could, asking nothing from anyone.

At the end of the show she laughed: "Turn off the TV kid. Let's go."

Smiling, Bette scooted to the door.

"I beat you Mommy. I'm ready first. Where we going?"

"Supermarket"

"Can I have a treat?" Wheedled the little girl.

'Hmm. You've been good. OK. We'll stop at the pet store and watch what's in the window." smiled Maiya. "Do you think it'll be puppies or kittens today?"

"Kittens. Hope it's kittens."

Jim Walters, unlocking the door, looked up and saw Bette skipping his way. "Hi." he said. "Want to hold a kitten while I get the box in the window ready for them?"

"Oh yes. Oh yes." came the excited reply. "Can I Mommy? Can I?"

Maiya said, "Sure." and grinned at her friend. Jim always treated Bette nicely. He was just a nice man.

Time passed while Bette hugged and kissed and scratched each of the seven kittens before handing them over to go into the window. Mr. Walters got the next hug and kiss. With Bette waving good-by, the two of them, mother and daughter, left the pet store and entered the supermarket. Bette liked to walk up and down the aisles on her own but within sight of Maiya. She didn't ask for anything but enjoyed the chance to choose things. "Let's get white bread Mommy. It's good toast."

With half a gallon of milk and a selection of fruits and vegetables from the mark down baskets, they headed for the checkout counter and then home with their two bags - a big heavy one for Maiya and a little one for Bette. Upstairs, Bette busied herself with her coloring book and crayons while the packages were unpacked and lunch cooked. Beans, salad, a slice of toast, and milk tasted good. Off came her clothes and she climbed into bed. Maiya followed her as soon as the dishes were done.

Mid-afternoon sun streamed in the window caressing their faces and waking them.

"Want the library or the playground?" asked Maiya. It didn't matter which Bette chose. Friends would be at both places. Friends for each of them.

The librarian read stories for an hour while the mothers talked. She spotted Jean - one of her favorites. Maiya listened and didn't add much to the conversation. It pleased her to hear the other woman's plans, what she would make for supper, which programs she would watch with her husband that night, the effort to get a babysitter for the weekend so they could go to dinner and a movie. It all sounded so normal, so different from Maiya's life. During the first couple of years after the birth of the baby while her mother cared for the child, things had been more conventional. Her job paid better and they afforded a restaurant meal once in a while. Tiredness didn't master her and most important - she had someone to talk to. But then, without warning, not even one day of not feeling well, her mother died. Life changed abruptly.

No longer able to pay for the larger apartment, she got a small one. That wasn't the main problem. Bette was the problem. Child care was the problem. She couldn't afford anything that she knew about. The city's free programs were full with long waiting lists. They added her name but gave her little hope. She needed work. Accepting charity, and that included welfare, was not something she could do.

Newspapers listed many kinds of jobs. Maiya read and thought about them all. Some sounded good. Once in a while she spotted one that looked like it would have a good paycheck attached. Some even said they were near good day care centers. All her efforts had a single result. Depression. She couldn't do anything. She'd only waited tables and that had work shifts. None of them were good for her.

Night after night uneasy sleep tormented. Waking up with impossible ideas, she'd cry herself back to sleep. But then, one night, she sat up in bed and excitedly thought: I bet that'll work.

Next day, with Bette beside her, she went to a diner and looked around before asking for the manager.

"Do you have an opening on the late shift? Could Bette and I eat our dinners here? How much do you pay? Are you busy? Will the tips be good? Do you pay my Social Security?"

She left her name and the manager said he'd call.

Driving ten blocks to the next diner on her want ads list, she parked and watched. It looks too good to be true., thought Maiya, busy street up front, parking lot in back, people going in and out. Maybe it'll work.

Swinging the car into the lot, she turned to Bette: "Out you go. Mommy wants to speak to the boss. I know you'll be good and not say anything. Give me a kiss."

The two of them walked around to the front and opened the door.

"Where's the manager?" she asked of the man who tried to seat them.

"Right here." he replied.

"I'm answering your ad." Maiya said softly, smiling at him.

"Is your little girl going to work too?" teased the manager.

"Oh no. I just brought her with me today. She won't bother you." and Maiya went through her questions.

All the answers were good. She liked the space. She liked the place. Mr. Abunda was pleasant and thoughtful. He got Bette a dish of ice cream and patted her head. Maiya watched him with the waitresses, the bus boys, the guys in the kitchen, the cashier. Everyone seemed to like him. Their attitudes said: We can tease. We can ask for things, but we'd better do what he says and be pleasant and efficient while we do it. This was the right place, so, respectfully, she asked for the job.

"I hope I suit you. I'd like to work here. You'll find I'm a hard worker." and her face and body language said *please.*

Abunda looked at her and thought to himself: I'll bet you will. You really want this job. Can't do better than that. "When can you start?"

Beaming, Maya almost shouted: "Tomorrow!".

That afternoon Mother and daughter followed the usual routine and she smiled when she saw Jean at the playground.

"Hey Jean. I got a job. Waitress in a nice diner. Boss is nice, too." and the two women pushed the kids on the swings.

A puzzled expression on her face, Jean said: "That's great. I know you've been wondering what you could do to make money. You like waiting tables. Maybe you'll meet a guy. Maybe this is the turn around for you. There's been enough bad luck. What'll you do with Bette?"

Maya stopped pushing for a minute. Should she tell Jean her plan? She didn't really know this woman? Could she trust her? No, she decided.

"Oh, I have a good place for her and I'll work the night shift so it's only while she sleeps. What's on TV tonight? This'll be my last evening in front of the tube for a while."

Always full of information and happy to share it, Jean thought and then answered: "That new crime show. You know, the one where the cops look at violence one way and the lawyers look at it another."

"Great. I like that one and I'll be too excited to sleep."

A little later Maiya took her tired little girl home and let her watch a bit of TV while she packed. Pajamas, toothbrush, slippers went into one bag. Blanket, container of water, pillow - went into another.

The pair made their way downstairs and over to the car. On the short drive to the diner Maiya went over her plans with Bette.

"I won't be far away. I'll stay 'til you're asleep and then come back to check on you a few times. Are you scared?"

Looking at her mother, Bette said: "A little. But it's OK. Don't worry. I'll be OK. And tomorrow I'll wake up in bed? Right?"

"Right." and Maiya hugged and kissed her daughter then got them both, and the bag, out of the car.

"Can I have meatloaf? I love meatloaf. And mashed potatoes? And corn? And milk?" Bette smiled at Mr. Abunda as she asked.

Smiling back, Abunda teased: "And ice cream?".

Dinner eaten, they headed for the restroom where Maiya helped Bette into her pajamas and watched her brush her teeth. After washing the child's face and hands, Maiya escorted her out, through the kitchen and out the back door into the parking lot. Their car was backed into the far corner. Quickly Maiya opened the trunk.

"In you go. Curl up on top of the pad. I'll put on the blanket. Did I bring enough pillows? Here's the water bottle. Remember I'll check on you in a couple of hours. You all right?"

And when the sleepy answer "Yes." came, Maiya closed the trunk. Leaning against the car, she listened intently. No sound. No whimpers. No cry. When her watch told her that ten minutes had passed, Maiya reentered the diner. Her mind whirred with worried thoughts. What would people think if they knew she locked her little girl in the car trunk? Would they think she was selfish to want to do things her way? Would they think she was indifferent to Bette's needs? Not concerned with her comfort? Distant about her safety? She had studied all the possibilities of child care. Nothing good existed for her. She couldn't afford to pay much and had no friends or relatives to ask for help. While she worked, her_attention was focused on one parking spot. Often at the back window she looked to see who was near the car. The first time it rained during her shift, she ran out and checked to see if the compartment got wet. It didn't. And as it got colder she brought a quilt to wrap the sleeping child in. Her scheme had to work. It had to.

Enough customers kept her busy for three hours and while her mind did go out to the car frequently, she managed to not show the anxiety she felt.

As the restaurant grew emptier she went to the night manager, Bill: "Good time for a coffee break? Need some air so I'll step out in the back."

Getting an iced tea, she made her way to the parking lot. Walking rapidly she was soon at the car. No one was watching her. No one was out there. The trunk lid popped open as she turned the key in the lock.

Bette was sound asleep cuddling her bear, with a slight smile on her face.

"So far so good." Maiya whispered into the night.

The rest of the night, the rest of the week, many weeks passed uneventfully. A new routine had been established. Maiya got tired but she learned to sleep when Bette napped and so could keep going. They didn't have lavish money but it was just enough to keep them going and put some aside. Bette was a growing girl and was about to outgrow her clothes.

Life went on.

Returning home, Maiya parked the car in front of the house in the early hours of the morning, got out, went to the rear, unlocked the trunk and picked up the child. Rough hands reached out.

"Give me the kid!"

Bette was pulled from Maiya's grasp and before she knew what was happening, her hands were forced behind her and she was handcuffed.

"Into the car lady."

She could see they were cops and the car was a prowl car but Bette was in another car and Maiya could see her crying as that car sped away.

"Where are we going? Why did you take my baby? Where is she going? Why is this happening? ..."

"Quiet lady. They'll tell you at headquarters."

And then she was standing in front of the desk. Bette was nowhere in sight. Maiya was terrified and thought Bette was probably scared too.

"Look lady, you've been arrested for child abuse. Why was that kid in the trunk of your car?"

Over and over Maiya explained her babysitting arrangement. Still the decision to take Bette away from her was made. Next morning, after the horror of spending hours in a prison cell, Maiya was given a lawyer.

Because she had no record, they released Maiya and told her to appear in court at the appointed time.

Despondent, she went to work that night. Bette's absence was a hole in her heart. Tears flowed easily. Food held no appeal. Tossing and turning in the bed at night, loneliness, fear of what might be happening to Bette, fear that she might never get her back, fear, fear, fear..... Days dragged.

Mr. Abunda stopped her as she came through the door. "What's going on? Where's Bette? How can I help? Tell me."

"Oh Mr. Abunda. She's gone. They took her. Said I'm an unfit mother. I'll never see her again." spilled out along with the tears.

"Come here." and he hugged her.

When she was calm, she told him the whole story. Explained her babysitting technique.

"I can't afford anything else and I want to support us. I don't want to take charity. I check her as often as I would at home. I look. Nobody sees me put her in the car. If she was sick, we'd stay home from work."

Thinking, troubled, Abunda asked how the police had found out.

"There's this nosey old lady who lives on the first floor. She's always looking out her window, spying on the neighborhood. She knows everything about everybody. I never thought she'd be awake at 4 in the morning but she must have been. She saw me take Bette out of the car one night and stayed up on purpose the next two nights. When she saw me do it again and again she must have thought I was doing bad things. I don't know what but she was sure I was taking bad care of my baby so she called the police. They came the next morning and caught me. What am I going to do?"

Abunda said: "Let me think. Go wash your face and get to work."

A few hours later, as she sat in a booth with a cup of coffee, Maiya was jolted out of her doldrums as a male voice said: "Are you the lady whose kid the cops grabbed?"

"Yes. Who are you?" questioned Maiya.

"I'm a reporter and it sounds like you've been unfairly treated. Tell me."

Headlines screamed: **CHILD KIDNAPPED BY COPS** ...and Maiya found herself famous. It was weird to see herself on the TV news. Strangers stopped her on the street. Some people cursed her and spat out their wishes that Bette be kept far away. Others praised her for trying her very best to care for her child. And then there was the woman who came to the diner with an offer.

"I live on the next block. I'm an old lady without much to do but I have an extra bedroom. All my children are gone and they almost never come to visit. I get lonely. Knowing a little girl was sleeping in the next room would comfort me and give me a reason to go on. Please can I help you?"

Maiya stared in disbelief. <u>Was this happening?</u>

"You care. You really care. But how do I know I can trust you? Bette has to be safe."

Mrs. Plotsky said: "Come to my house tomorrow. See how I live. We'll talk. Meet my neighbors. You'll see."

In a week the two women went to court. Maiya's lawyer met them there. He had been told of the new development. Reporters were there. The judge listened intently, saw the hope on Maiya's face, Mrs. Plotsky's arm around the young woman's shoulders, and thought of all the children who had been returned to truly abusive parents. Give this one a chance. went through his mind.

"I will return the child to this mother on the condition that she report back to the court in three months that her child care responsibility is fulfilled in a more conventional manner. Young lady, it is my opinion that your little girl is blessed to have a mother who cares so much. Good luck."

Later that day the three of them, Bette, Mrs. Plotsky, and Maiya, sat close together in the diner's booth and had ice cream before going to visit Bette's new night time home. As Mr. Abunda joined them, laughter, talk of the past and of friendship crisscrossed the table, filling the air with joy.

A recurrent theme in Barry's writing concerns the long-burning fuse of anger about to explode in a child abandoned or abused by a parent. In this chilling 1993 story, a serial killer is unmasked as highly atypical.

SUBWAY

Tuesday, October 9th. For the first time in a year it was a woman who died under the wheels of the subway train. The last death had occurred in September.

Scurrying up the stairs that morning, Lucille was filled with sad thoughts. Poor man. What a way to end your life - beneath the wheels of a subway train in a grimy underground station, attended by a host of uncaring strangers who were shocked for the moment but would soon forget.

Flashes of elation sparked amidst blue feelings in her head. He doesn't have to go on. Life is over for him. No more problems. He was young. Maybe things were going good. Maybe he died happy. And so, smiling gently to herself, Lucille emerged from the kiosk, walking sedately to the bus stop.

No one noticed her. She was not noticeable. Under the frumpy clothes and unbecoming haircut, an attractive woman hid. A pleasing image, if not a beautiful one, lurked beneath the surface. Her shape wasn't Marilyn Monroe quality but the breasts were firm and thrust upwards, the waist had a moderate dimension, and the appealing derriere was small, plump and firm. All was secreted under a shapeless skirt of medium brown and a tan shirt without distinction. The beige cardigan she wore had neither graceful features nor pizzazz. Plain, low brown pumps covered her feet and the hemline of her skirt concealed the contours of her legs. A watch with large, easily read face and a pair of small gold earrings were Lucille's only jewelry. Her purse was big enough to hold sandwich, apple and paperback. If a stylist had cut her hair with even slight regard for the dimensions of her face and neck, the result would have been appealing. A little makeup could complete the job. A good looking woman would be the result. But remaking the exterior wouldn't instill the self confidence and self respect needed to carry off the new appearance. She had lost those years ago, as a child. *Child. I wonder if that little girl is happy? She looks happy, crossing the street on her way to school. But you can't tell from the outside. Nobody ever thought I was unhappy. I'd like to ask her but here comes my bus. Maybe I'll see her again.* Boarding the bus, Lucille noticed activity around the subway entrance. Three patrol cars and an ambulance, lights flashing, cluttered the street. Seeing excited people crowding around, some annoyed, probably at the delay in getting to work, she thought: *I'll read about it in the evening papers.*

Thinking ahead, Lucille always left home early to make sure she got to the department store on time. Though the trip was much longer on the bus than on the subway, the morning's incident didn't keep her from arriving a little before nine. Clocking in, she went straight to her post. Towels were her merchandise. Selling them was easy. Few customers had questions more profound than: "What are they made of?" She had neatly stacked the goods the day before, no new supplies had arrived, and there were no special sales in her department. As she checked the displays, the day seemed to stretch ahead uneventfully but that was fine. It gave her time to relive the morning's events. Some of her coworkers noticed that she seemed a bit happier than usual, a little more outgoing, a little less concerned with herself. "Hey, Lucille, let's eat lunch outside today. You look like you're having a good day, I'll bet I even saw you smile. What happened? What's making it good for you? Tell me while we eat."

While they ate, Ann, who worked in the next department, wondered why her invitation to brown bag it together was so quickly accepted. But she couldn't get answers to her questions. The woman on the bench next to her just smiled serenely and shrugged. Lucille felt the warmth of enjoyment spread itself across her body and mind. Mentally hugging herself, she enjoyed the brief walk they took. "What a beautiful day. I love the fall. Look at that blouse. Isn't it pretty. Too much money but I'd love to have it." The window shopping brought her pleasure. Already, clothes for next season decorated the mannequins posed behind the glass in a variety of awkward, graceful stances. "Come on. It's time to start back." Lucille insisted, typically, that they return a few minutes early. Afternoon time went by quickly and pleasantly. As the work hours ended she found herself humming quietly.

In the supermarket, after getting off the train, she shopped for a treat for dinner. Frozen dinners were too expensive so she didn't even consider them. She didn't like them. They didn't give her enough to eat. Lack of appetite was not one of her complaints with life. She debated with herself: *Should I treat myself to lamb chops or a really good steak? Ummm. Steak, asparagus and a baked sweet potato. That's good. I'll enjoy that and after all, I deserve it.*

As usual, at this hour of the day when working women shop, the aisles were crowded and the lines at the checkout counters were long. After paying for what she needed plus a few other things, scouring powder and tissues, Lucille headed home. Climbing the flights of stairs to her apartment at the rear of the old brownstone, she remembered finding the place ten years ago. *It's too expensive for a one bedroom flat,* three *floors up, probably roach infested*, she thought. *It needs paint. But it's got a newly tiled bathroom.* Excited at the idea of being on her own, she put down the two months deposit and was given a key, her key.

At the age of twenty-two it signaled escape from her parents. The job at the department store (had five years really passed?) was not her first and now she had saved a nest egg. *I can make it. I've never let myself down. I can do it. I can leave home. I can get away.*

"If you go, you can't come back." were her father's encouraging words. "You'll miss me. Maybe I'll come to see you."

"Don't. Don't come to visit me."

So she had left without giving them her new address, carrying one suitcase with the few things that mattered to her and her meager wardrobe. When she got a phone she would call and give them the number but she never wanted to see either of them again. Parents. There must be good ones in the world but her's sure weren't. Memories of childhood were not pleasant, were positively horrible.

Did everybody have that kind of growing up?

She remembered when it had started. She was seven or eight. That part wasn't clear but being invited into her father's bed was. He had said, "Mommy's working and I'm lonely. Come, keep me warm." And she had. A job as a waitress kept her mother away from home through the supper hour and late into the night. The two of them, father and daughter, were left alone. He made the meal, usually not a very good one, and saw that she did her homework. When bath time came he often fussed with a warm, sweet smelling tub of bubbles for her and watched her pleasure in the drowsy, dreamy, soaking atmosphere. Gently toweling his little girl dry, he slipped a nightgown over her head and led her to her bed. Until that night when the routine was prolonged. She had fallen asleep, been awakened by a gentle hand and drowsily agreed to his request. Later that night he carried her back to her own bed, kissed her and tucked her in. Five nights a week her mother worked and five nights a week Lucille fell asleep in her father's arms.

It had not been a big bed, just a standard double. The bed in the apartment made that other one seem shabby. King-sized, canopied, seductively draped in pastel flowers and silken sheets, it was the only piece of elegant furniture she had and the only one she wanted. It was her one indulgence. Every day she changed the expensive linen, plumped up the many pillows. Even with Lucille's store employee discount it cost a good amount to keep the bed richly covered. She lived under the canopy, reading romance novels, watching television, eating breakfast and dinner there, indulging her fantasies. There was only one bad memory. Try as hard as she could it wouldn't go away.

At first, on her own, Lucille didn't attract men but the day came when one of the guys at work asked her out. Twice they went to the movies. On the third date they ate dinner in a small, neighborhood restaurant and then headed for the apartment. Her sexual dreams were about to come true. He held her and a chill swept down her spine. As his head rested on her breast a feeling of uneasiness possessed her. When his mouth caressed her nipple, horror engulfed her. Desperately she pushed him away. Suppose he tried to..., tried to... The strength of fear allowed her to break his grasp. Chocking, gasping, she managed to blurt out: "LEAVE ! GO AWAY ! Just go." Bewildered, he did.

Sobbing quietly, she stripped the bed and made it anew. No real flesh and blood man would ever lie on it with her again. It was *her* bed. There would be no pain there as there had been in daddy's bed. Memory surged over her and she hugged the pillows. His hand between her legs had brought her out of slumber and when he entered her the electric shock, the agony, made her faint. Waking a few minutes later she found him caressing her lovingly. The words mocked the movements. "Don't never tell nobody. It's our secret." And so it remained.

She had tried to tell. When it got bad, when she knew it was wrong, she had needed to let her mother know.

"Ma. I've got something to tell you. It's important."

"Not now, Luce. I'm pooped. Let me sleep for a bit. Then we can talk. My feet are killing me."

Years went by. Fifteen years to be exact. Her hate for him expanded into a hate and fear of all men. They were ugly, hurting beasts. She had done the world a service that day ridding it of one more. That made three.

Method had been carefully imagined. *I'm not smart but I figured that out good.* Lucille grinned to herself and felt great satisfaction when her plans worked so well. Always waiting for a crowd, she'd find the one small man who was eagerly leaning over the subway platform at the sound of the approaching train. A slight shove and over he went. Continuing the upward thrust of her arms she covered her mouth and screamed at the terrible thing that had just happened. Turning, she gazed at the others and made her way to the stairs. It was a good way to start the morning. It made her day happy, upbeat. Treating herself to a special supper, she eagerly waited for darkness.

The smooth sheets, the slight whisper of air over her nakedness, her own gentle hands twisting and caressing, the release after the crest of fulfillment, all made her cuddling, curling sleep totally satisfying. Waking with the sunrise, she was ready to begin the day.

Articles in the morning paper never hinted at the possibility that the murderer was a murderess. It never occurred to the detectives or reporters. No large woman had been noticed at the scene of the crimes and no-one had ever recognized that the victims were all slight men. That was a secret she could hold to herself.

Weeks passed. Lucille, feeling ill tempered, crotchety, knew it was time to cleanse herself and the world once more. She took her usual train four stops to a station that was not familiar. Moving to the part of the platform closest to the stairs, Lucille looked around. There was a nice crowd and yes, there he was. Carrying a briefcase and jacket, he looked a little anxious, deep in thought. From far away in the tunnel came the sound of an approaching train. Almost as if to confirm that it was a train and not some other strange apparition, he leaned over the edge. Lucille put up her hands and stepped forward pushing her body toward him. At the last instant he twisted and stepped to one side.

"Oh my God!"

"That poor woman."

"It was so fast. Somebody call 911."

All the witnesses swore that she had been shoved. Their descriptions of the murderer varied but they all were positive - she had been pushed.

Barry took courses in creative writing. As one of her assignments, she was to tell a story with an unexpected component. Reaching into some remembered New York experience, Barry converts the stress of needing a bathroom into an unforseen though delightful victory.

A Funeral

Oh Shit ! she thought. I've got to pee again.

The problem had been Kate's as long as she could remember. Here she was, trapped in the middle of the afternoon, on Madison Avenue. Madison and where? she wondered. At the corner the street signs spelled out "Madison" and "82nd St. " No department store in sight. No restaurant in sight. In the past, in big stores, she used ladies' rooms without making explanations. At other times she ordered as little as a cup of coffee or a Coke in a restaurant and headed for the loo.

Stopping in front of a store window, she sighed and opened her purse. Zipped into the little side pocket was a folded set of papers. Opening them and scanning quickly, she found the heading which covered this neighborhood. There it was: "80th - 85th Madison Ave." Listed was one restaurant on 80th Street and a funeral home on 81st.

The list was started five years ago and kept up to date frequently as she added items. Kate loved walking the east side avenues and came in from the suburbs at least once a month to indulge herself. Blonde and petite, her forty-five years showed neither in her face nor in her figure. Buying little from the boutiques and small expensive stores Kate thoroughly enjoyed herself window shopping and investigating the shelves and racks. For years, when the kids were young, she hadn't wanted to be away from the house when they came home from school. Now Jim was at college in Boston and Ann was a senior in high school. No longer needed at home at 3 o'clock, the entire day became Kate's. When she came into the city, the supper she had cooked the night before needed only to be heated up and added to with a few last-minute trimmings. Her daughter and husband would not feel neglected.

An image of her husband flashed into her mind. She loved him. Smiling to herself, she remembered his typical teases during their engagement: “A bathroom again? You just went an hour ago. I can't take you anywhere without planning ahead to find a john. When we're out in the woods I've got to scout up bushes for you. Remind me never to take you fishing.”

One evening he had gotten furious. New business possibilities were being discussed with that night's acquaintances. “Goddamit!” he whispered savagely through clenched teeth. “I'm just setting up this deal. Why the hell do you have to interrupt now? Cross your legs!” They were standing on a street corner in an elegant section of a town in which she was a stranger. There were no hotels or restaurants in sight but it didn’t matter. She couldn’t go to a diner or coffee shop in formal clothes and ask for the ladies’ room. Kate waited as long as she could and then decided breaking into the conversation was better than leaving a puddle on the sidewalk. She spoke up. Embarrassed, they returned to the house where the reception was held. Years later they could laugh over the incident, but for a long time Curt thought that he lost a good investment because of her.

Another memory flickered. It took her back to her teaching days. She continued to work after they married and counted as one of her blessings the fact that her classroom was right next to the teacher's room. Assigning the kids an absorbing task, she could slip out and take care of herself before she was missed. Only the occasional day during the summer or Christmas vacation, when she and her friends went into the city, gave her trouble. They were an understanding crew, and usually there was at least one other as desperate as she. Big stores, museums, or fancy restaurants were their targets, so she did not find herself without facilities as she had that night with Curt.

Getting caught without a john at hand could happen again, but not, if she could help it, on an east side Manhattan street. She started the list in an offhand way but then ritualized its construction. Her habit was to explore the city systematically, so she thought of its geography in terms of a grid whose boxes consisted of five short numbered blocks and two long avenue blocks. One section was just right for a day's walk. If she felt particularly energetic or if the stores were nonexistent, or, uninteresting, she might do two grids in one day.

Always, the day after her city expedition, sitting over breakfast coffee, when all the other occupants of the house left, she carefully added notes to the list.

Nice little hotel, she mused, but a little too small to let me parade through the lobby unnoticed. Hmm. I'll put it down anyway but asterisk it so I remember to use it only as a last resort. There were three restaurants that would do. She chuckled to herself and wrote down the maternity store two door from the corner. They often had bathrooms, open to their pregnant customers. She could fake it. She remembered how it felt. Even as she thought about it her bladder began to feel full. It was an old familiar strain. "Urgency" the doctors call it. Good name. It was worse when she was pregnant. The pressure of the baby made it almost unbearable. Waking up in the middle of the night, after the baby was born, was not new for Kate. Now she had two things to do -- go to the bathroom and feed the baby. However, she was now back in the present.

Rising from her chair, she headed for the small, half bath next to the kitchen. It had been convenient for the kids when they were small and always handy for her. On the walk back to the table she thought about the pretty blue pleated dress she looked at in the maternity store and wished for a second that she was pregnant and could buy it instead of just using it as an excuse to head for the store's bathroom. Back to my notes, she thought, there are other things to do today besides this.

Her mind slipped back to yesterday, and, in her imagination she was once again standing on the street, bladder full.

Looking down at the list in her hand, she noticed the funeral parlor was closest to where she stood and she needed something close. It was impossible to walk with clenched knees, and she would soon be at that stage. Folding the papers and reinserting them in the bag's zipper compartment, she began moving downtown. Aah. Kate saw it across the street. She walked past the school which occupied an entire side of the block, got to the corner, waited for the light, and marched across. Quietly she entered the front door.

Her eyes looked left and right. After spotting the female profile on one door, her glance took in the other doors. Display signs directed toward two funerals. There was a medium sized crowd milling about at the entrance to the first viewing room. No one stood outside the other. Quickly she entered and found the sign-in book. One name was inscribed. When her eyes adjusted to the dim light she saw the male figure in a front pew. She couldn't guess an age. His hair was gray, but the face he turned to her was young, smooth. Nodding he turned his attention back to the closed coffin and seemed lost in thought. No expression had crossed the features. Was he sad? Would "What's his name" in the coffin be missed? Kate's questions had to go unanswered. Her bladder was well past the "full" mark. Using the attached pen, she wrote her name, address, and a short sentence --- Fond memories. Turning, she trotted out of the room, across the lobby, and into the toilet.

In a split second she was emptying herself. A sigh of relief escaped her lips, and a contented smile fastened on her face. Pulling up her panties and rearranging her clothes, she left the cubicle, washed her hands, and departed from the melancholy institution. Maybe she was the only happy person walking through its doors. Glancing back, she felt glad it existed.

Kate strolled through the rest of her grid enjoying the galleries and art shops. She loved watching people. Some strolled, some hustled, some were chic, and some were shoddy. On Fifth Avenue, across from the museum, a young family sauntering down the street, amused her. The young mother pushed a stroller containing a three year old. The young father, wearing designer sports clothes, carried a leash. At the end of that tether was a very small tricycle. Brilliant idea crossed Kate's mind.

That evening, when she was telling Curt the details of her day's activities, she didn't think to include her funerary expedition. She kept the details of her list private. It was nobody's business. She was tired of being teased on that subject.

Weeks went by occupied with the usual round of things to do. She met her friends for lunch, went to the gym, swam, supermarketed, read, wrote letters, made dinner, and took care of the house plants and garden. Pleasantly busy, life slipped by.

Returning from the market one afternoon, she was fumbling with her keys when the phone rang. A package spilled across the table and the door gaped open as she grabbed the receiver and breathed: “Hello?”

“Mrs. Baker?”

“Yes,” she said, hoping it would be a short conversation. As usual when she got home, she had to pee.

“You don't know me, but I am the executor of Mr. Flemming's estate.”

“Who? Who did you say?”

“Mr. Flemming. According to the terms of the will you have inherited half of his possessions. I will need to meet you to make arrangements and to have you pay your share of the funeral costs.”

“Mr. Flemming? I don't know any Mr. Flemming. You must be mistaken.”

"No. I don't think so. William Flemming. You went to his funeral on May sixteenth."

"I'm confused. I don't remember any funeral. Where was it held? How did you get my name?"

"Let's see. Oh yes. It was at the McGuire Home on eighty first and Madison. You signed the book."

Softly, timidly, she said, "Yes. I remember now."

"Well, according to the terms of the will, the estate is to be divided among the mourners who attended the ceremony. When can I see you?"

They made appointments. Name, address, and phone number of the lawyer were recorded. After hanging up the phone, Kate peed, unpacked groceries and started supper. Humming to herself she went upstairs to dress in the outfit Curt liked best. Coming down, she set the table. Smiling inwardly while she put out wine glasses, Kate thought: It's nice there's always a bottle of champagne in the refrigerator.

When she heard his car in the drive, she lit the candles and dimmed the light in the dining room. Curt unlocked the door, stepped across the threshold, and looking around, quizzed: "How come we're not eating in the kitchen? What's going on?"

"Because I love you." Throwing her arms around his neck, she snuggled for a second and then held him at arm's length.

"Let's go on that dream vacation we've been talking about for years. You know, Paris. My treat."

Surprising, Hitchcockian, chilling, disquieting are adjectives to describe the gruesome events in this 1993 sad story of an unending search for love. Barry reveals depths and thoughts that could not be imagined by family or friends. In her words: "My story tells of a young man who had been given away at birth. His life is filled with an inability to integrate the truths of his life into a normal existence. The solution he chooses for his problem, is the crime. The love he finally finds comprises the final tragedy."

Ma

The witnesses walked soberly from the viewing room when the execution was over and the prisoner pronounced dead, all but one. She rested against the cold wall. No tears flowed down her cheeks. She didn't reach out or talk to anyone. A glance told the guards, the priest, that she was deep within herself with a "No Visitors" sign hanging above her head.

It was over. He was gone.

The beginning seemed so long ago - theirs and his. Birth is the start for all of us and for him, tragedy began then, when he entered the world. As he grew, he became aware. He had no parents. No-one loved him. He wasn't special.

Through all the seasons of the year the orphanage encircled Robert and defined his world until at the age of four, he went to the first of many foster homes. They were all awful, demanding of him things he couldn't give and giving things he couldn't accept. "Family life" was outside his experience. He knew it existed. He could see and feel and almost smell the warm rich earthy aura surrounding the families passing through his world, but the *how* of *how to do it* was beyond understanding. Wishing for it grew, and made life in a family that he couldn't accept as his, hard.

Looking across the room at each other, Robert and Max lit up inside. Here they were, again back in the orphanage together. Across the supper table they glanced at each other, grinned when no-one else was looking and knew that night would bring talk.

Just <u>talking</u> was hard for Robert. Usually he listened:
"Pay attention and you'll grow up to be a good man." foster father number five spewed out.

"Go to school. Keep your room clean. Do what your mother tells you. Say your prayers. Come to church on Sunday. Don't steal. Don't fight with your new brothers and sister. Get your chores done on time. And don't eat too much."

No warmth. No affection. No hugs. A demand for a goodnight kiss which he dutifully placed on the cheek of the woman sitting in the living room chair. None came from her.

A schoolyard fight over the usual taunts boys throw at new, foster kids, developed.

The principal's call explained: "His shirt is torn. He's dirty and he has a bloody nose and black eye because he was in a fight. The other boys tell me he punched first. Please discipline him. We can't have that kind of behavior."

Robert wouldn't answer the questions his foster mother flung out into the room. Punishment. More chores.

A shouted: "No new shirt. I'll fix this one."

Ridicule came from the other kids at the supper table. And he hadn't even won the fight.

He didn't do what they wanted but his table manners were good. He was hungry. When they started sending him away from supper, Robert exploded, fought with everyone, stole money to go to the hamburger joint.
"We can't live with this. Back you go. Wrap up your things. I'm taking you now."

And so, he was in the orphanage again.

Max's case was different. After a couple of months his parents always came for him. When all the money was spent and they couldn't feed him they'd bring him back. So here he was.

Luck was with the boys. They were assigned to the same dorm. Promises to hand over desserts for a week got them beds next to each other.

"Lights out!" was called.

Impatiently the two waited and then began to talk. Max was sad.

"Wish there was more money and I wasn't the kid they chose to give away. Why can't they send Ruth or Bill? Why me? How long this time? It's hard to keep up in school and I wanna graduate High School so's I can get a good job. I'll always have food for my kids. I'm 12 now. Think I'll make it?"

Robert listened.

"Sure you'll do it. You're a good guy. At least you have a home you come from. Parents. Where'd I start? What's my mother like? Everyone's got a mother so I know I had one. Why didn't they love me?"

He turned on his side pretending sleep. Nobody would see him cry - ever. In Robert's head the thoughts kept coming back, circling, tearing at him. *Where was I born? They told me when I was born so I know how old I am. Fourteen. Who do I look like? Do I have brothers and sisters? Is her house nice? Does she bake cookies? What's it like to sit at a table and be loved? What's it like to be loved? What does a hug feel like?*

The night passed and he woke up angry, sassed Ellie when she put the food on his tray, ate everything in front of him and tumbled the tray to the floor.

"Not me. I ain't cleaning up no mess."

...and wound up in the supervisor's office.

"You can't keep up this behavior Robert. What happened this morning to set you off? I've asked but nobody has a clue. Talk to me. Help me understand you. What would you...."

A teacher flung herself into the room.

"Come quick. There's been an accident."

"Stay here Robert. Think about what I said. I'll be back soon."

Robert looked around. The plain, meant-for-work office had been opened for the day. He smelled the soap used to scrub the floor. Light slanted in through the shades. A fan circled slowly, humming. Filing cabinets, desk, closet were unlocked. *Wonder what's in my file?* Scrambling over, he looked.

That night he told Max.

"They know who my parents are and where they lived when I was born. They weren't married and he left her when he found out she was gonna have a baby but she gave his name on the papers she had to fill out when she gave away her baby. When she gave *ME* away. Maybe she didn't even hold me. Not even once. The town was small. Nobody wanted to adopt a kid so they brought me here. This place is home. Max, I hate it. Going to run away and I'm gonna find them Max. I'm gonna find them."

Four years passed. There were no more foster homes. He was too old for that. As he approached eighteen he gained good control of himself. Rules were followed, school was attended and indeed he was about to graduate High School, assigned jobs were done. To others, wirey, blond Robert appeared quiet, withdrawn, without friends, cool. Reality would expose a boiling, never quiet, self-concentrated, brain full of thoughts, angry thoughts.

"Happy Birthday Robert. How does it feel to be eighteen? Feel grownup? You look grownup. That'll help you when you look for a job. Eighteen is our top age, you know. When school's over you'll have to leave and go out on your own. We'll help. We'll give you a hundred dollars to start with."

Walking away from the set of buildings that were the only home he ever knew, he felt a little lost, certainly friendless (he had last seen Max a year ago) but determined and free.

Now, what comes first? he thought. *Job, place to live, phone book, meal? JOB! I can live for a while in that old abandoned shack on the Will's place. Not for long but until I get my first paycheck.*

"Hey. What's the best paper to look for a job?", he asked the clerk in the candy store.

"Well - here's the town paper and this one lists government jobs. You gonna stay around here or try the city? If you're going to the city take their daily rag. Take 'em all and decide later."

He bought them all.

What kind of a job can I do? I don't know how to do nothing, came into his mind. *I'm not big enough to do a real hard job but I can carry and I can file and I ain't stupid. I can learn what they show me.* And so, feeling rather "up" he took off.

"Already hired somebody."

"I don't think you're right for this position."

"Come back tomorrow."

"Yeah. OK Go to the office and fill out the papers. You can start on Monday."

YEAH. OK. START MONDAY. YIPPEE.

And he treated himself to an ice cream soda when all the forms were filled, when he knew where the time clock was and where his card would be. He knew where to report Monday at 8 and who to ask for. He had an idea of what he would be doing. Life felt good.

The luncheonette wasn't full so he planned to use it as an office. At the 5 & 10 Robert bought a small notebook and ball point pen both blue, his favorite color. Back at the restaurant he sat at a bigger table than he thought he was entitled to, ordered a glass of milk and piece of strawberry shortcake and asked to borrow the phone book.

His father he found easily. The house was on Gardner St. in a nice but not ritzy section. His mother's name wasn't listed. After puzzling over her absence he realized that she had probably gotten married. Next step was the town record office. He knew what year to start at. His birth year. Marriage records were kept forever so all it would take was patience and patience he had.

Life, 'til today, had been unlucky but luck was with him now. He only had to read through a little more than 2 years of records to find the listing of her marriage. Now he possessed her new name and her husbands name. It was enough. The phone book gave her address: 192 Elm Drive. Ironically, it was just a few blocks from where his father lived.

I wonder if they ever see each other on the street or in a store?, he mused. What do they say to each other? Do they smile? I know one thing they never talk about - ME. Robert's mind settled back into it's usual seething turmoil. He smiled at the waitress as he returned the phone book, left the luncheonette and returned to the old shack where he was living. Not much to look at, it would do for another couple of weeks. Work would start in three days.

Monday came. At 7:45 he arrived at the time clock. Yup, there was his card. He punched in and went to look for Fred.

"You sure you're strong enough to lift heavy boxes? Maybe you're too skinny. Don't your Ma feed you enough?"

Robert still smiled although he had taken an instant dislike for Fred.

"Try me. Think you'll be surprised."

Fred was.

"OK kid. Put these cartons on a dolly and take 'em to aisle 6. That's where canned vegetables are. Open a box, stamp the price on top of each can with this stamper and put them on the shelves. Each shelf has a label with the name and size of the can that belongs there so it should be easy. You can read, can't you?"

"Yup."

And the day began. When it ended he walked over to the bus garage where buses from all the routes were taken care of and got a map showing the town's bus stops. Then he headed for the luncheonette and had supper. It was a long walk back to the shack but his mind was busy so it seemed quick. Now he knew how to get to Gardner St. and Elm Drive. Sleep came easy that night, deep, satisfying sleep.

Leaving work at four, he strolled to the corner where #16 bus was scheduled and sure enough, there it was. Six stops later he transferred to # 3 and rode twenty minutes. Getting off three blocks before Gardner St. he walked casually past the house, registering the terrain in detail in his head. Woods behind the house were meager but if he laid on his belly no one would spot him and he would be able to watch as long as he wanted.

Planning, Robert decided to observe “Daddy” for a few weeks. He savored future time when “Mommy” would live under his scrutiny.

“Got a good used bike? Let me see that blue one, Don’t take out that one. The tires are no good. Yeah. I like this one. How much? Oh come on. Fifty is too much. I'll give you thirty.”

Land extended out behind his supermarket. Overgrown land, used for nothing, unappealing. He took the bike there and easily found the cover he had fashioned for it from black garbage bags and strapping tape. The bike would be his means of transportation out to the observation points. Cheaper and faster than the buses, it was an inconspicuous vehicle. People in the neighborhood would get used to seeing him - a kid on a bike. He never rode it near work nor near the room he had rented. Nobody who knew him should mentally connect him and the rundown blue bike.

Work wasn't exciting even though he'd been taught to use the forklift and do jobs in the warehouse. Theirs was the storehouse for all the chain's outlets in the county, so huge stacks of goods were in the large space. Now he was in charge of rotating the goods so the freshest were at the bottom. He also took the cartons of things to be shelved by the stock clerk, to the doorway.

He was doing just that when it happened.

The forklift, piled high with stock was rolling toward the doorway when he saw the kid dash in front of him.

“Watch out. Get out of there. Move.” he shouted as he jammed on the brakes.

The machine stopped. Cases came tumbling down pinning the boy to the wall. Parents yelled. Robert jumped down, grabbed cartons and sent them crashing every which way. Soon the child was free, crying but unhurt. He was a little one. Maybe four years old.

Mommy picked him up and comforted: “Hush Nicky. You're all right. You shouldn't have run away. I've told you and told you - stay near the cart.”

Daddy was speaking to Robert. “Thanks. If you hadn't stopped in time we might have had a mess. He shouldn't have run into the warehouse but you know kids. They always do what they shouldn't. Are you all right? You sure tossed those boxes around. How can I say 'Thank you'?. I know. I'll go get another steak and you'll come for a barbecue Sunday.”

Sunday came. Wondering what it would be like, Robert made his way to the Hendrick's house. From the outside it was a cheerful place. Painted yellow it had white curtains in the windows and flowers he thought he could smell from far away, in a border and circling a big tree on the front lawn. A note was taped to the front door. Come around back. Robert went.

Half way around the house, he heard the laughter.

“Be careful. You'll spill it.” chuckled the woman of the house.

“Hi Robert. Glad you could come. Nicky say 'Hello'. Come on you can help me. Go into the kitchen and bring out the potatoes. They're the things wrapped in aluminum foil on the sink.”

“Good job. Now, while those are cooking we can play a little catch. Robert, Nicky, over here so we won't knock over the grill. You've got a talent with the ball, Bobby. Can I call you Bobby? Your father must have played with you a lot. I love ball, any kind of ball - football, softball, baseball, soccer, basketball... Hope Nicky likes it. It's a great way to spend time with your son. OhOh. Marge is calling. Bet it's time to set the table. Follow me.”

And set the table time it was. What a meal. Robert had never had one like it. Fresh made fruit salad, baked potatoes, corn on the cob (all you wanted), steak, salad, bread and butter, and at the end - chocolate chip cookies, home made chocolate chip cookies. Nicky acted like a kid. He made too much noise and jumped around at the table. Marge corrected him, lovingly but strongly.

Five o'clock came and Robert went home. Sitting in the comfortable chair he had bought, he thought over the afternoon. The warm feelings, the sharing, the love all seemed so natural to these people. How strange it was to him. Maybe some day he could have it in his own life but first, first he had things to do.

For two weeks he watched. Nobody noticed him. The small pocket of trees was sufficient to hide him. Once, when the kids were playing ball, the ball rolled toward his lair but he put his head down and the boy and girl didn't discover him. "Dad" was a dull man with little variation from his usual patterns. Robert's half brother and sister were equally uninteresting except for the fact of their existence.

At seven o'clock on that Thursday evening, Robert stepped out of his hiding place and approached the man putting garbage in the can.

"Well Hello."

"Hello Dad."

"Dad?"

"Yes. DAD. I'm the kid you forgot about. I'm the one you made before you got married. I'm the one you walked out on before I was born. Thanks."

He took out the knife and with all his force, with all his hate, he plunged it into his father's chest. The look of surprise, the look of horror on the older man's face would stay with Robert and please him all the rest of his life. Remorse, guilt, sorrow did not exist.

Pulling the knife out, he wiped it on the piece of rag he had brought with him, and strolled back to the bike left in the bike rack at the small mall a couple of blocks away. Before riding away he threw the rag into the dumpster at the end of the row of stores.

No one had seen him. There had been no noise. Probably many minutes would pass before the family realized daddy hadn't reentered the house. They would go looking for him. Robert didn't think it had happened yet. He heard no sirens. Whistling, he rode back to the supermarket and put the bike in its place. The walk to his rooms was pleasant. He stopped on the way and had supper in the luncheonette. The meal was good. Meatloaf. He loved meatloaf. Portions were big here and he had all he could eat.

At home he took out the knife. No blood was visible but he wanted it like new, shiny, menacing, for the next time. Lying in bed that night, he smiled. The best part would start tomorrow. Her. He would see her.

Get to know her. Watch her. Sleep came.

Maybe luck would be with him and he would see her but No, she wasn't outside the house and there was no car in the driveway. Next day the same thing. Three more days. His timing must be bad. Perhaps he should come earlier, or later. OK. A new week would give him a new start.

Monday morning he called in sick: "It's nothing very much, I just want to rest. See you Tuesday."

There she was. There she was. Plump, short, carefully coiffed blond hair, dressed in slacks and a ski sweater she got out of the car followed by three girls aged (he guessed) four to twelve. One word that seemed to fit her was "soft". Her body looked soft, good to lean against, comfortable to curl up to. Her attitude toward the children was soft. She didn't shout or use a harsh voice. She laughed and smiled.

He only became aware of where he was when the foursome entered the house. It was time to leave his position across the street. Time to peddle back and put the bike away. At suppertime he wasn't hungry and made himself a peanut butter and jelly sandwich at home.

Sadness, depression swept over him. It would have been nice living with her, growing up in a house like that. Oh how he hated her. How much he would enjoy killing her. What would she say when he talked to her? What look would be on her face when she died? Where would he do it? When?

During the next few weeks he followed her, tracing her paths, learning her ways. She often went food shopping at night when her husband was home to watch the kids. The supermarket parking lot wasn't crowded in the evening. That would be the place. That would be the time.

Anxiety crept into his head. The pleasure he had anticipated wasn't there but determination remained.

She was in the store. It was 9:30. The bike was lying in the uncut grass near where her car was parked. He lounged against the black Ford parked a few spots away. Waiting.

He must have closed his eyes for a few seconds because he had missed her leaving the store. The grocery cart rolled toward him and then stopped at the far side of her car. It was the side away from the lot. She opened the back door and began putting heavy bags on the seat.

"Hello Ma."

"Hello who? What do you mean Ma? I'm not your Ma."

He laughed. "Oh yes you are Ma. It's your fault you've never seen me. I was there. You knew where I was. Bet you never thought about me. Know you never cared. I'm that baby you gave away. Hello Ma."

"Oh my God. I thought..."

"Yeah. You thought I'd just disappear. But here I am and now I'm going to kill you. Ma."

"Please. Please..." and she crumpled to the concrete.

He yanked the knife out of her chest, walked over to the bike and rode away.

When he finally got home he realized he was shaking. It was over. It was finished. Now there really was no hope. She would never come for him. Never.

The headlines next day screamed "Second Baffling Murder". The story mentioned that both victims had been stabbed but there seemed to be no other connection between them. Yes, they had gone to the same high school but were in different years.

Robert felt complacent. He would never be connected with those people.

But he had forgotten Max.

Max still lived in town. He was a shoe salesman. There was time during the day to read the newspaper. He read. Something troubled him. He had heard the man's name before and - wait a minute - the woman's maiden name. Where? Thoughts rumbled around in his head for a few days. Then he went to the police.

"Sheriff, I know who did those murders. I don't know where he lives now but you probably won't have trouble finding him. Maybe the orphanage knows where he is."

"Why?"

"Because they were his parents. That's why."

Surprise poked through his depression when Robert opened the door and saw the two policemen, guns drawn. He put up no resistance. Armed with a search warrant, they easily found the knife. Robert hadn't thought to hide it.

The trial was fast. Conviction was anticipated and so it came to pass. The sentence was also not unexpected. He found himself on death row.

Days passed endlessly. Slowly he began to realize he didn't feel well and when he couldn't drag himself out of bed, he asked for a doctor. They took him to the infirmary and then to the civilian hospital. They took him in chains. He was put in the intensive care unit. A cop sat, out of the way but as close to his bed as possible. Gradually he became aware of the nurse.

She was gentle. Caring. She knew his name. What was hers? How could he find out? IDIOT. Ask.

"Iris".

She wasn't beautiful. Neat. Clean. If you can say it about a person - comfortable.

They began to talk. She told about her life, her family, her love of nursing, her pleasure in helping people get well.

And then he was moved to a private room. Different women took care of him.

Soon after the shifts changed, Iris came to his room. With the cop just outside the door, they had half an hour together. It seemed a lifetime. It passed too fast. As he woke in the morning, he smiled at the idea of seeing her that afternoon and was disconsolate when they put him in a wheelchair and announced their destination as the prison infirmary. He had lost her. He would never have a friend.

Blue, he existed in the infirmary uninterested in whether he was getting better or not. Just lay there. Did nothing. No books. No TV.

"Robert. You have a visitor."

"Visitor?" Who would come and see him?

Iris walked in.

"Iris".

He didn't know whether to laugh or cry. He did neither. Just looked at her.

She, however, laughed.

"Here's a chocolate bar I thought you'd like. It was easier to carry than chicken soup. Aren't you going to say 'Hello'? Never mind. You look so much better. How you feeling?"

"I wasn't feeling so good but now that you're here I'm fine. Was it hard for you to get in? How often can you come? What will people think - you visiting a guy in jail?"

"Never mind other people. It's you and me who're friends."

Weeks, months, a year passed. Gradually he began to talk to her, told her his feelings. Let her know his deep losses, that feeling of being left out. Robert spoke of his longing to have a mother, to be a family, to be loved.

"You are now. I love you and I'm old enough to be your mother. Let me. I've always wanted a son."

Robert refused to appeal the sentence. He had committed premeditated murder and the orphanage had taught him well. Each person is responsible for their own actions. Do something and live with the results. His parents had.

The day came. They had arranged for Iris to be in the viewing room. As the lethal dose was administered, Robert turned his head to the window and mouthed: “I love you.”, and then he died.

Submitted for competition to the National Writers Guild in 1997, this 1995 grim short story shows another aspect of Barry's thinking. It is difficult not to attribute the genesis of such a sad life-ending tale to worsening diabetic complications. Alternatively, the subject change could be based on maturation as an author.

NOT LUCKY

Pete's wife looked at him sleeping in the hospital bed. Calmness marked the features but she knew that would change when he awoke. That, however, was not what concerned her. Lucy occupied the front of her mind.

Maybe it would be different if there were more children to share the burden but there weren't. Lucy was the only one that had filled the pretty white crib. Now she was all grown up, living on her own. Problem's fell on her shoulders almost as thick as dandruff. Toxic Shock Syndrome had pushed sickness into her life and while the doctors declared her cured, the tiredness lingered on.

Perhaps the lack of animation in her walk, the slight dragging of her feet, the lack of interest in the people around her, made her muggable material. So, mugged she was. It was a vicious crime. The big man grabbed her purse yanking it with enough force to break two fingers. She screamed and he took that to be defiance. Not one to be defied by a little woman, he slapped her face and shoved her off the curb. Lucy's bad luck held and her right leg was gashed open by the smashed glass in the street. Hours spent in the emergency room of a big city hospital, found her discharged into her own care, needing to get home but without money because that and her keys were in the stolen purse.

As the awareness of what could be waiting for her in the apartment, dawned, tears started to flow. Like a little girl she said: "I want to go home."

No-one was listening.

Feeling around in her coat pocket the finges on her good hand searched for coins so she could call home. Dirty tissues and a bus transfer shared the space with one dime and six pennies. None of the people in the lobby seemed prosperous and Lucy had never begged before, but now was certainly the time to learn.

"I was mugged and I need nine cents more to make a phone call so they'll come and get me. Please, do you have some change?"

New York has a reputation as being cold and hostile but the generosity of the city showed through. Before she could turn around or even say "Thank you." her hand held eighty-four cents. It was more than enough.

"Ma. I got mugged and I'm scared to go home. Can I come stay with you? Will it be all right? Thanks."

One bus would take her there and it stopped only 2 blocks away. Maybe her bus transfer would get her on. It was today's. Evening was coming and Lucy was afraid of being out, alone, in the dark. Feet don't drag when you're in a rush and her feet were no different. Swiftly they carried her to the bus stop and to her delight, a bus, the right bus, was just down the street. Keeping herself under control she handed the driver the official form and sighed with relief when he took it. Maybe her luck was changing.

Thirty-some-odd blocks later, Lucy descended the step, stood on the corner and gazed down the block. During the last years of her life here, the apartment house seemed dirty, unappetizing, cold, but now it was an old friend of a building, declaring itself anchored to the sidewalk. Almost running, Lucy got to the door, swung it open, crossed the dim lobby, and pushed button 3 in the rickety elevator. Twelve steps took her to her parent's door. Quickly it opened and she found herself in her mother's arms.

"Come in. Come in. Take off your coat. Now why are you crying? You're here. Want a cup of coffee? Come into the kitchen and tell me what happened. You're hurt. Your leg. Your hand. Do they hurt?"

Between sobs, while gulping the hot coffee and asking for a piece of cake, Lucy did her best to repeat all the trials of her day. Exhausted but comforted by the old surroundings, relaxation took hold. Startled when the door opened, Lucy's muscles tightened. It was Daddy. Like a little girl, she rushed over and threw her arms around him.

He stroked her hair and shushed her sobs. Like Mommy, he told her: "you're home, you're safe. Now tell me what happened."

Still shaking, she described the mugging. "He was so big. I tried to hold on to my purse but there it was, in his hand. My fingers hurt so much. I yelled. He cursed me and shoved. Why is there always broken glass in the wrong place? Maybe some car got broken into here. Anyway, it cut me. Blood started to run all over the place. Somebody had called the cops and they came pretty fast. They wrapped something around my leg and put me in a patrol car. On the way to the hospital they asked me all sorts of questions. I thought I could identify the man so they drove me around looking for him. We didn't find him. At the hospital the doctor stitched up my leg and put splints on my fingers. They said I could go home but it popped into my head that that man had my keys and my address. "I'm scared" I thought. "I don't want to go there." I begged for money in the lobby. Can you imagine me begging? Well, I did. I got eighty-four cents and there was even a quarter so I called you. Oh, I'm so glad to be here. Didn't someone say: "Home is that place where they have to take you in."?

Lucy and Pete both called work the next day and asked for a personal day. Next, Daddy went to the bedroom and searched for the extra set of keys to Lucy's place while she searched the desk in the living room.

"Here they are.", called Mom from the kitchen. "They were in the junk drawer".

Digging around in her old closet, Lucy managed to find some old slacks and a shirt. Putting them on she declared herself ready to go.

"Come on then", said Daddy and off they went.

The subway was not particularly pleasant but they felt no sense of menace. That was left for when they approached the apartment door.

It was closed. Daddy gingerly tried the doorknob. He couldn't turn the knob so he knew the lock was holding. Inserting the right key and doing all the right turns, he opened the door. All lights were off. Listening, he decided nobody was inside and cautiously stepped in. Nothing looked disturbed so he called out: "Lucy. Come on in. It's O.K. You have to check and see if anything is missing. I'm going to call someone to change the lock. Where are your yellow pages?"

They picked a locksmith in the neighborhood ut were told the wait would be a couple of hours. Walking to a neighborhood restaurant for lunch, they laughed at each other and said how glad they were yesterday was over with. Tuna sandwiches eaten, coffee drunk, they strolled back. Without thinking, daddy inserted the key and opened the door. Inside, Lucy headed for the bathroom.

She heard the thud and quickly exited the john. Daddy was on the floor. Blood poured from his head. Looking up she saw the brute she would never forget. Her favorite bronze statue was in his 12 hand. Raising it above his head he moved toward her. The last thing her mind was aware of was the woosh of air as it descended.

The locksmith found them. Lucy was sprawled backwards in the chair, dead. 911 responded quickly. Soon a phone call brought the wife who was no longer a mother, to the hospital. None of them was lucky.

Using only 850 words, Barry in 1995 creates the imagery of tragedy. Was the spark for this idea generated when she (Barb for Barry) sat in the car while her husband (Ed for Eli) aided an injured cyclist?

A ONCE QUIET ROAD

Motorcycles. There were five of them shattering the quiet of the narrow road. Barb and Ed drove along enjoying the beautiful New England fall colors, the sense of solitude broken only by the occasional car hustling past. A feeling of threat, a sense of evil, radiated from the cycles. Noise crashed across their senses. *Will we die?*, thought Barb. The couple looked at each other.

They next met at the traffic light. “Come on man. Race me.” Waving wildly, hunching his shoulders, gunning the bike, the leader challenged the man in the car who pointedly ignored him. Tossing their heads, hooting in derision, the group roared off. The girl behind the front driver looked back at them.

“Weaving back and forth across the road like that. Daring me to race. I hope we don't meet them again”, Ed complained.

“But they're only kids. Dumb kids. None of them are wearing helmets. Not the boys. Not the girls. I'd be afraid to ride double like that. I'd be afraid to ride, period.” retorted Barb with a frown on her face and fists clenched tightly in her lap.

Ahead, the road once again stretched quietly.

A soft breeze soothed them as they traveled the winding road. They forgot the cycles. Forgot until they saw a massive scatter on the road far in the distance. Soon they made out figures standing around, spilled bikes, the pickup truck facing the wrong way in the intersection, the sprawled body on the macadam.

Ed jumped out and ran to help. Excitement, control over people's lives, adventure, being a hero - all made his existence as a doctor, a great real-life all-consuming exhilaration. Barb sat in the car. She could do nothing to help. Blood didn't scare her she just didn't want to be in the way. In a while Ed would come back proudly announcing: “I saved that kid's eye. He's got a couple of broken bones and scrapes and cuts but the eye was the bad thing and I think I saved it.”

But that was in the future. Time passed. Her mind wandered.

Where was the girl who'd been riding with the guy who was hurt? She wondered about her, not knowing how close to the truth her imagination brought her. All the girls looked alike. Stringy streaked blonde hair pulled back into pony tails, bodies that were no way voluptuous but thin and unimaginatively dressed in jeans and T shirts with unimportant, say nothing logos. Sneakers completed their uniforms. She could see them ten years from now - blowzy, sloppy fat, a tooth missing, scruffy kids hanging on their legs. *Why were they out riding with these guys? What did they want?* The answer was simple - *love.*

Barb could guess what their lives were like. Lisa - Barb invented a name - was probably typical. Seventh of ten children, she had been neither oldest, nor youngest.

“You ain't the prettiest or smartest but at least you didn't get F’s and you ain't cuttin school. Gimme the card. I'll sign it.” snarled her tired overworked mother.

And so she did. Pops was either not home or too drunk to care about this middle girl. As she grew older Ma’s comments changed.

“Why ain't you in school more? You won't get a job if you don't pass in school. What'll become of you? You'll get to be a hooker and that's not good. The church says it's a sin.”

There was no "Get to your room." There was no room to get to. She had the outside spot in the bed (not enough blankets) with four sharing. No place for her things. No privacy. No sense of worth. Life was a drag.

It was easy for Barb to imagine Lisa and her friend sitting on the steps and talking: "*Hey, did you see Meg today? That old skirt was her sister's. Don't she ever get nothing new? You babysitting Saturday? Guess they won't let you have company? Going to give all the money to your Ma or keep some for yourself? Keep some. You earned it."*

Reality. Today's problems. No dreams.

Then Mike came along. "Hey girlie. Want to ride on my bike?"

"I'm scared." she screeched but he laughed and showed her how to get on. She went. Her arms around him made her feel secure. Drinking beer in a bar with the rest of the gang brought a sense of belonging.

"Don't go with that guy." Ma warned but there was no where else to go. Defiance made her feel better.

"Try to stop me." Lisa shrilled back and was gone.

A figure stepped from the woods. The girl's knock on Barb's car window startled her. A look of desperation, of fear, of being lost bathed the face that stared in. *"Oh my God. Is she hurt? What do I do?"* welled into Barb's mind as she opened the door and swung out with open arms.

"Hold me, Lady. Hold me."

Letters and Commentary

Barry was a vocal partisan for all matters impinging on the welfare of diabetic kidney patients. These four letters — the last written six months before her death — illustrate her sustained effort to focus the American Diabetes Association on the daily life of diabetic people.

July 27, 1993

Jean Whalen
Director, Government Relations
ADA National Center
1660 Duke Street
Alexandria, VA 22314

Dear Ms. Whalen,

It is difficult for me to find words to describe my reaction to your letter of July 20, 1993.

My point is not to change the labeling of insulin vials. The metal caps that hold the stoppers in the bottles can **easily** be marked with large indentations or bumps to signal to the blind or visually impaired which type of insulin is being manipulated. Dr. Kessler of the FDA assures me that the FDA does not regulate this part of the packaging and that its design is up to the manufacturer. He further tells me that the FDA would quickly give its blessing to such a change.

I therefore, now request that the ADA put its power into urging the manufacturers (Eli Lilly and Novo Nordisk) to institute such an improvement in packaging. Please note that this might cost a few 29 cent stamps but not the vast amount of money you refer to.

The ADA is still claiming to work for the improvement of the daily life of the diabetic. I urge you to live up to that pledge.

Sincerely,

Mildred Friedman
President
Diabetic Renal Transplant Self-Help Group

August 30, 1993

Dr. James Gavin
President
ADA National Center
1660 Duke Street
Alexandria, VA
22314

Dear Dr. Gavin,

I read with interest in *Diabetes Care* (16:1051, 1993) of your ascent to the presidency of the ADA. Congratulations.

The statement attributed to you that "ADA has to be responsible for appropriate interpretation and application of the DCCT results...", delighted me. I am fearful that the results of this important study will be misinterpreted and misapplied. I base this on everything I have read (with the exception of the report in *Diabetes in the News* - an Ames Co. publication).

1. Reduction and slowing of microvascular complications of diabetes by an average 60% is significant, not conclusive.

2. The full range of diabetics were not included. Minority populations were poorly represented as were the older patients.

3. Severe hypoglycemia is usually not defined as happening in the middle of the night. Loss of consciousness is underplayed (to my personal trepidation - I have been on the floor for 12 hours). Frequent lack of symptoms accompanying daytime low blood sugar is often not mentioned.

4. Significant weight gain which can sabotage the program is not thoroughly explained.

5. Necessity for screening to eliminate those patients who should not try for tight control is insufficiently stressed. Endocrinologists will probably handle this well but the general practitioner may either not be aware of it or not practice it.

6. And last of all is the failure of the DCCT, even with its high degree of compliance, to achieve euglycemia. It is my belief that the 40% difference between realized blood sugar values and wished for blood sugar values, is in the same category of importance as the 60% reduction in complication rate.

In other words - caution, caution, caution.

It is my wish that your term in office be filled with great advances and good for the diabetics in our nation and the world.

Sincerely,

Mildred Friedman

Nov. 12, 1993

Dr. James Gavin
President
ADA National Center
1660 Duke Street
Alexandria, VA
22314

Dear Dr. Gavin,

I have received no reply to the letter of which I have enclosed a copy.

Let me quote from the **first** paragraph of Dr. PiSunyer's Presidential Address as published in volume 16, pgs. 1521-25, 1993 of *Diabetes Care.*

The Mission of the American Diabetes Association is "to prevent and cure diabetes and to improve the lives of all people affected with diabetes."

I take this to include the blind and visually handicapped. Please explain to me why my logic is in error.

Sincerely,
Mildred Friedman
President
Diabetic Renal Transplant Self-Help Group

March 5, 1997

Philip E. Ryer, MD
President
ADA National Center
1660 Duke Street
Alexandria, VA
22314

Dear Dr. Ryer,

Four years have passed since my last letter to the ADA. The problem has not been corrected, indeed, it has become potentially worse. A new fast acting insulin increases the risk to the blind or visually handicapped diabetic. The ADA did send a very gentle letter to the manufacturers with no results.

Isn't it time that the ADA got behind the patients and created a storm?

Sincerely,
Mildred Friedman
President
Diabetic Renal Transplant Self-Help Group

Like so many other attempts to further her cause, Barry's really sound concept for improving the utility of eye glasses was left without response. She did not, however, give up or give in and persisted in trying to change — for the better— how we do things.

July 2, 1996

Leonardo Del Vecchio
President Luxottica
LensCrafters
P.O.Box 429580
Cincinnati, OH
45249-9580

Dear Mr. Del Vecchio,

Like many of your customers, I wear a pair of glasses hanging around my neck. LensCrafters has provided me with great glasses for many years. It's the hanging part that doesn't work well but I have an idea.

Building the hanger into the glasses frame should work. It would be an extension of the ear piece. In this way the "peeper keeper" would not slip off and would not break at the metal connection. I would suggest starting with a line of half glasses incorporating my innovative design.

There are new ways to look at old problems.

Looking forward to hearing from you,
Mildred Friedman

A further example of Barry's campaign to make insulin use easier for those with impaired vision.

February 21, 1994

Ed Bryant
Editor
Voice of the Diabetic
National Federation of the Blind
811 Cherry St., Suite 309
Columbia, MO 65201

Dear Ed,

Forgive my procrastination. Please.

Here is the pertinent correspondence.

Let me just point out a few things. Dr. Kessler called me personally to inform me that the packaging of insulin, **except for the metal band that holds the stopper in the bottle**, is under FDA regulation and that if we can get the manufacturers of insulin to in some way mark those bands, the FDA would give its immediate blessings. I asked for a brief note in writing to confirm what he had told me. I was assured it would be in the mail shortly. Still waiting.

But the second part of my story is more devastating. These people who earn their livings on the back of diabetics have a poor understanding of the terrible complications of that disease. Nowhere did I suggest the use of braille. Those who have lost their sight and kidneys probably suffer bad neuropathy and a loss of feeling in their fingertips. Suggesting color coding for the blind is, at the least, ridiculous. Yes, there are aides to fill syringes but that doesn't help to tell the vials apart. Aaargh!

I also wish they had learned to adequately read English. My statements are quite clear.

Do what you want with these but let me make a request. If you publish them please send copies to the higher ups in the ADA, Eli Lily and Co. and Novo Nordisk.

Thanks,
Mildred Friedman

After bilateral vitreous hemorrhages caused by proliferative diabetic retinopathy, Barry became blind with vision restricted to counting fingers at two feet. After partial reabsorption of clots permitting limited ambulatory vision, she began a desperate quest for an ophthalmologist who might improve some of her sight. In this short essay, Barry notes how an eye specialist may overlook an obvious necessity in patient care.

On Going Blind (Sometime in 1977)

Gee that's a pretty rose but watch the thorns.

Once we've learned how we take for granted our ability to read. The brain doesn't forget the skills but if the eyes go wrong that doesn't matter.

I find myself surrounded by little pieces of paper - letters, notes from children ("I'm at the store"), instructions, telephone numbers, cleaning slips to choose between, receipts - each one demanding a response. The magnifying glass is picked up, faint printing worried through, a problem solved, the slip put down and then -- hours later, not recognized - to be mulled over again. Others can't be blamed they haven't been here but lordy, lordy don't save recipes for me or send me cards.

The eyes hurt, I become afraid and reach for my connection to the one who will reassure me. Hunting through the piles of paper I find at last his business card. Dr. --- ophthamologist, ### Park Avenue and over in the corner his number - too small to read.

Dimitrious Oreopoulos, a personal friend, did not escape Barry's constant energy dispersal directed at forcing attention on the patient. Asked in 1995 to assist in continuing the journal Humane Medicine, Barry pointedly advised the editor that patients require empathetic attention as well as the health care team.

To: Dr. D.G.Oreopoulos
Editor
Humane Medicine
Fax 416-603-8127

From: Mildred (Barry) Friedman
1049 E. 17th St.
Brooklyn, N.Y. 11230
Fax: 718-252-3718

October 5, 1995

I have been mulling over the Memorandum concerning the future of *Humane Medicine*. While it points out its concern with input from the concerned medical community stressing the need for communication in two directions, it does not seem to include the one group that justifies its existence. While you speak of the trend to depersonalize caregivers and caregetters and treat them as commodities, you do not treat the latter group at all.

In both Canada and the U.S. patient groups exist. Patients are intelligent and certainly involved people, in the issue of patient care. You seem to have fallen into the trap usually occupied by hospitals: the least important group is the patients.

I would suggest that you reach out and include them.

Barry pursued her noble heritage visiting cousins directly descended from the original Barrett-Lennards. There were title holders and even castles somehow associated with her past. In this 1980 letter, Barry seeks to combine her quest for self-identity with her new profession as a writer.

1049 E. 17th Street
Brooklyn, N.Y.
February 15, 1980

Scott McDade, Editor
Family Heritage
P.O. Box 1809
New York, N.Y. 10001

Dear Mr. McDade,

The enclosed is true but it tells little about me as a person. I am a forty-four year old woman in pursuit of a fourth career.

I was born and spent most of my life in New York City. Due to the circumstances we were poor and a college education would not have been possible if it were not for the city universities. Thus I obtained a Bachelor of Science from Brooklyn College where I also met my future husband. As an aside he has submitted to much kidding for changing my name from Barrett-Lennard to Friedman. I worked for several years at Kings County Hospital as a bacteriologist and parasitologist before moving to Boston and becoming a laboratory technician at Harvard Medical School. I stopped working to raise my three daughters, then switched to teaching after returning to school. I taught the youngest grades at a public elementary school here in Brooklyn for ten years. My retirement is forced by a number of medical handicaps including loss of vision which explains this size type.
I am currently trying to establish a new lifestyle. It must be one that allows me to work in my home. Perhaps it will be writing.

Yours truly,

Letters and Commentary

Mildred Friedman

Even life-long friends were fair game when benefit to patients was Barry's objective. Here like the shoemaker's children who have perforated soles, Barry calls Peter Lundin to task for lagging behind in bringing the influence of the American Association of Kidney Patients (AAKP) to bear for Brooklyn's kidney patient population.

March 5, 1994

A. Peter Lundin, MD
President
AAKP
1 Davis Boulevard, Suite 302
Tampa, Florida 33606

Dear Pete,

This is a hard letter to write but the subject is one that has troubled me for a long time.

Let me get right to the point. There is no AAKP presence in the dialysis units of Downstate. I have not visited the Kings County unit but my guess is that there is none there either. I do not know about your unit. The Renal Clinic has none except for that which I supply.

I do not understand how, as president of the organization, you have allowed this to come to pass. Born in these hallowed halls, nurtured here at its beginning, it now occupies a vegetative state. The mission is to serve patients. In order to do that, patients must be reached. The updated membership package which arrived on my doorstep, is lovely. The available publications are probably worthwhile, energy spent lobbying for renal care is valuable, but the kidney patients I speak to have never heard of AAKP.

Something is missing. Something is missing in your home ballfield.

Sincerely,
Barry

Concise yet to the point(s). Barry conveys just what is involved by the request that a diabetic perform fingerstick blood glucose monitoring. Somehow, I feel guilty reading what is actually prescribed.

On Being A Human Pincushion

Pincushions come in many sizes, shapes, and colors. There is the standard American red one kinda shaped like a pumpkin with a dangling strawberry connected to the stem place. That little berry is filled with emery so pins and needles pushed into it and moved around, get sharpened. It just occurs to me that I don't know what's inside a pincushion but I'm sure not going to cut one open to find out. Slipper shapes, with pincushion stuff where the foot is supposed to go, flash into my mind. Then there's the wrist pin cushion used by professional seamstresses. And then - there's me.

Oh yes, I am truly a pincushion. Probably pierced more frequently than pincushions which don't belong to people who sew for a living. You see, I'm a practicing diabetic. Doctors and other members of my Health Care Team tell me I've got to keep my blood sugar level in the normal range and that in order to do that three insulin shots a day and a minimum of three blood sugar checks each day, are called for. Easy for them to say. I get to be the pincushion.

Serious diabetics test their blood sugar level 30 minutes before breakfast, before lunch, and before dinner. This knowledge is used to inflict discomfort. It lets you "informed guess" how much insulin to take to handle or cover the amount of food you expect to eat. Don't get me wrong - insulin injections are not painful (except for that once in a while when you've chosen a sensitive spot). Now. Count. Three times a day. By bedtime, you're a pincushion.

OK. You know what an injection is. Pushing a sharp pointed thing through your skin and squirting in the medicine. Now learn how to do a blood sugar test. Examine the words: BLOOD SUGAR TEST. You guessed it. Blood is needed. There's no way you can talk yourself into bleeding. Hypnosis doesn't work. Commands won't do it. Only contact with another sharp pointed object will do the job. Lancets fit the description but it's hard to point them at your finger and jab. Usually the puncture is too deep and it almost always hurts, which, unless you're an idiot, will make you think twice about doing it the next time. In an attempt to ease the lives of patients (I'm giving inventors the credit for being good samaritans) devices have been designed which hold the lancet. cock it, and then shoot it into the flesh held under it. The depth of the stick is controlled and is not very deep. Comparatively painless pricks are the result. Fingers are usually used although toes and ear lobes are also possible.

Let me tell you quickly what happens to the drop of blood you've just bled. Put on the reagent pad (a piece of paper that has special chemicals and is held by a surrounding strip so you can carry it), it is allowed to act with the chemicals for a specific amount of time like one minute. After that the color change of the reagent pad is either read by a machine or in other varieties of strips, by your eye. Now you know your blood sugar value.

This whole affair intrigues my grandchildren. Once while I was visiting my four year old granddaughter, she put me on display. Her best friend was visiting too and like me, was invited for dinner. I took out my supplies and heard Ruthie excitedly whisper to her pal: "Wait 'til you see what **my** grandma does!"

Three meals a day. Three finger sticks. Here I am - the human pincushion. Those six skin punctures are only a minimum number. If your sugar level was high, you'll do another one two to three hours later and if the value isn't down, watch out, here comes another dose of insulin given, as you've learned, through the skin. Low blood sugar levels don't call for another shot but tell you to eat some sugar. "Goody," you say but who wants a chocolate bar at four in the morning?

Here I sit before you (I write at a computer), a pierced individual, a Human Pincushion. Pity me not - but don't expect a great outpouring of sympathy when you tells me: "I don't like needles." I don't either.

I'm told that on the drawing board is a device that can shine a beam of light through a finger and tell by the amount of light that is absorbed, the blood sugar level. My fingers are smiling in anticipation.

Actually finding proof that the family stories told her as a child were true source of joy for Barry. As a result, she ultimately traveled to Australia, England, and Canada to meet wonderfully receptive cousins.

Strange Heritage for an American

As long as I can remember I've known that I was noble. There was a depth in playing "princess" that existed because of a real connection to castles and kings. My story is jumbled because it is child-hood's memories made real in middle age. Let me begin not at the start nor at the end which has not yet happened but in midstream, a few years ago.

On my first visit to England, like many tourists, I went to the British Museum but unlike the others I brushed past the Rosetta Stone, mummies, signatures of monarchs, Elgin marbles and the rest to head for the library and its section on nobility and family histories.

Without too much difficulty I found a brief description of that group whose name I had been born with, whose name my mother was the last bearer of in New York City and perhaps in the United States.

A crest, a motto (Pour bien desirer - to wish well), seemed to leap off the pages at me. A history of generations followed. My grandfather was listed as an emigrant to Canada; his daughters were lumped in a sum, four, no names given; his sons, in order, with their occupations. My father came second. Hardinge Barrett-Lennard, spelled perfectly and next to it one word, gentleman. "You lie". I said out loud "He was no gentleman!" and turned away, hurt again by my contact with him.

He had married my mother when they were both past forty. They had met aboard a ship traveling to England. He had visited his grandmother and not taken his fiancee with him. She had wondered later if it was because she was a Jew but then learned from him long afterwards that it was because he was doing the old lady out of some securities. No matter, after fathering two children he left her.

Contrary to what Debrett's printed he was an unskilled laborer who did not like to work.

Through all the years that followed he chose not to contact his children but he had left behind stories of a titled family. I grew up hearing of how his father's generation scattered to the colonies because there were so many of them. I heard the words Sir and Lady, knew a vague story of a castle on the Thames sold and demolished about the time of the first World War. Heard of a sister whom he had loved but not stayed in close touch with.

I knew he had come from Vancouver, B.C. and that his mother had died shortly after his birth, that there had been a copy of a family history destroyed by mice while we lived on a chicken farm, but little else.

While I struggled with a hyphenated name that I was somehow proud of, I was also ashamed not knowing the people. I grew up feeling repulsed by the lack of contact. I felt unwanted. So that first meeting in London with their reality pleased and disturbed me. When we returned home and I told my mother about what I had found she brought out a signet ring I had never seen. My father had given it to her many years before but she had kept it to herself. The motto was there. The crest was there. Now it was mine.

For years I did no more about the Barrett-Lennards. My children grew up and summer vacation became something I could plan without them. My husband had a business date in Seattle in August and suggested a trip through the Canadian Rockies. "Could we go to Vancouver?" I asked and was told "Sure." Thus I found myself in a hotel room, sitting at a table with a phone book in front of me staring at two listings:

Barrett-Lennard, Walter Jr.
Barrett-Lennard, Charles

They had to be family but how would they react to me, a stranger, a Jew, a daughter of my father? Shaking I picked up the phone and dialed the second number. A woman answered.

I explained who I was. She was my aunt by marriage. My uncle had died a few years before, the last of his generation. Yes, she remembered my father, she was in touch with his nephew (my first cousin) who had been best man at his wedding. She gave me the name of another first cousin and his address. She was warm and friendly inviting me over for a visit. Tears were so close to the surface that I told her this contact was enough for now, that I would write.

I did and received a package containing the Debrett's information, a description of a church connected with the family (Chelsea Old Church) and enclosing a family monument (the Dacre Monument). There was a story about the family mansion, Belhus, which was described as being associated with the Thames, currently in decay, ungraced by water, and remarkable more for its size than for its architecture. Belhus was mentioned in a deed written in 1397. She mentioned the possibility of a visit to Brooklyn with a copy of that family history mentioned before. Time will tell what that conversation brings.

After the first phone call I settled back, collected myself and dialed again. Another female voice, another explanation, and another invitation. This one I accepted and that evening met my first cousin, his wife and one of their children.

Yes there certainly is a title, a baronetcy, held now by a priest and to be passed next to another priest of a different faith. Neither will have an heir so the question is where after them. My cousin is in touch with a few other relatives in Canada and with a large branch of the family in Australia. I haven't contacted them yet. Turns out that the family history was printed for the males in my father's generation and that he has his father's copy. I couldn't see it, however since it was not yet unpacked from their recent move. So near and yet so far! A fascination with our joint past sparkled in his eyes and led to hours of told story. There were tales of regiments started for the crown, of Barretts and Lennards, of Queen Elizabeth I and good friends whose names you've read in history books. My mind whirled and wouldn't keep it straight. I was enchanted by his man who looked so lordly there in his armchair in a modest home in Canada. He welcomed me to the family and it mattered not that he was a tax collector and I was a schoolteacher. We had this touch with history.

We talked of British Columbia and he told me that an ancestor of ours had been among the first to circumnavigate the island of Vancouver, that the old boat (the Tempter) had just disappeared during his lifetime and that a book describing the journey was about to be reissued.

I left, a future of discovery ahead of me, a warm feeling about the Barrett-Lennards in my heart at last. Months later there will appear in the Manhattan phone book two Barrett-Lennard listings, one for me and one for my sister, just in case someone is looking. But the best part of all was calling that sister as soon as I got home and hearing her reply to my "Well, we are noble." "oh, Oh, OH!".

Religion was anathema to Barry. Although morality, charity, and justice were major controlling forces in her life, a belief in a superior being was not. Surprisingly, clergymen of several denominations regularly interacted with Barry in multiple roles. The Barrett-Lennard "title holder" was a catholic priest who flew the Atlantic to celebrate Barry's 10th and 15th kidney transplant celebrations.

No Miracles

There are no miracles. Long years ago when I realized there was no God I leaned on people giving up the mysterious forces some believe in.

I did not expect then the lightning and thunderbolt kind of happening. I wanted only someone to care and listen. I hope I have learned now not to even want to bare my soul much less try to do so. My complaints are a long and tiring list. They have been called a litany of griefs. For all those medics who get tired of listening I will try to cease my lists but I do hope they remember that doesn't stop the hurts and discomforts. It doesn't make the aches Andeans go away because they are not said.

I am not a round peg for your round hole. One of us is square. No matter which one.

Too much was expected of this new doctor. That was my fault. I have seen him twice in 3 weeks. During the interval I did everything that I was asked. The second time he decided to control my out of control diabetes. Great! I don't want to be whacked out with high blood sugar. He did ask me how I was. Gave him 2 problems to start him easy. Told him of my bad headache of the day before and that my bad eye was still bleeding. To satisfy himself he looked in I hope it did him good. He proceeded to put me on a 1200 calorie diet to loose weight and control the diabetes. Sounds great but one day on the diet I had another stroke, my good eye bled, my blood pressure went up and I started to gain weight. So far I'm up a pound and a half.

The world is receding from view again. I can't see traffic lights and walk signs.

My husband, who has come home to cheer me up is asleep on the couch and I have taken more Valium. The depression he feels is my fault. All I wanted was a doctor I could tell. I do not want to be a file for them. I want to feel better.

> *Barry applied for top notch writing courses. Evident in Barry's responses to questions is the breadth of her interests as shown by magazine subscriptions which included: National Geographic, Vanity Fair, Gourmet, Lear's, Family Circle, Woman's Day, Archaeology, Biblical Archaeology, KMT, Smithsonian, Natural History, Writer's Digest, Diabetes Forecast, Living Well with Diabetes, Diabetes, Diabetes Care, Diabetes Self Management. Other responses provide insight into Barry's psyche.*

Tell us who you are?

In April, 1992, Barry described herself as *"a free lance writer with an MS in education who is 56 (and happy to be there) and married. My interests are: cooking, handcrafts, traveling, reading, archaeology, Egyptology, autographed document collecting, grand-mothering, reaching out to other patients as a professional patient myself."*
"I have written and had published magazine articles, a short story, and columns for 2 patient organization periodicals which deal with diabetes and diabetes and its complications. Short stories and the one novel that is in my head, greatly interest me as future writing expressions. I regularly read: novels, magazines, newspapers, poetry, publications for patients, and medical literature."

Why are you interested in writing?

"As a child, like many children, I wrote poetry. It was not a driving force in my life but a satisfaction resulted. Time passed. Education, marriage, motherhood, disease - all took turns. As an academic physician interested in diabetic kidney disease, my husband was asked to find several patients to write a column for a Canadian kidney patient magazine. He suggested two other people and ME. They never got it going but I've been doing it for four years.

There it was - my name in print! I was hooked. Then it came to me. Writing medical things is fun but I really wanted to tell stories. And so I do but there is room for improvement.

Demonstrate that you can you think like a writer.

"Sue could feel the knot in her stomach. Her hands tensed. But she smiled and relaxed her face. If it was within her power, he would never know how his words affected her. Neatly dressed, without makeup except for lipstick, smelling of her favorite perfume, and with a good dinner ready for the table she refused to acknowledge his verbal abuse knowing that it would play itself out - again. Years ago she had given up arguing and decided to handle him this way. It kept her sane."

Tap into your experience for a writing concept.

How to become a human pin cushion

1. Acknowledge that you must become one, that you are diabetic and face the necessity to know your blood sugar level.
2. Wipe the tip of your finger with an alcohol swab and shake it at the floor to dry and pool blood in it.
3. Put a new lancet in your lancet holder. Remove the cover. Cock it (lancet holder, not the cover).
4. Place the lancet holder on the cleaned finger - hard. Fire the damned thing.
5. BLEED Squeeze your finger from the palm of your hand to the tip until there is a nice round drop of blood.
6. Being careful to not ruin the drop, turn the blood glucose meter on and insert the test strip when the meter instructs you to.
7. When the meter reads "apply sample" put the blood on the white circle in the strip.
8. Use the alcohol pad to put pressure on the spot that was bleeding.
8. Wait.
9. Read your blood sugar value when the meter beeps two times to tell you that it has finished.
10.Put your equipment away ready to use next time you must be a human pin cushion.

Focus on a subject to write about

The little boy at the snake zoo.
Telling the death of your baby.
Four years old and watching your father leave.
Hunting for your four year old who wandered away while you were on a ferry trip.

Chose one subject, give it a title and write it.

But Not a Small Child

It had been a wonderful safari. Walking up to a herd of wild elephants was an experience I will never forget. All my senses were alive when the mass of zebras thundered by in a swirl of dust, hooves pounding, voices braying, leaving a pungent smell in the air. Experience followed experience. Africa.

Lion kills, leopards in trees, salt licks, watering holes, animals, animals, animals, birds by the score but no snakes. Not a single one did we see.

It wasn't a serious complaint but still we wanted to see a reptile. And so, when the game viewing was over and we were back in Nairobi we chided the leader about our disappointment. "OK" he said. "This afternoon you're off to the snake zoo. Just one favor. Can my four year old son come with you?"

The taxi ride was short. Paying the driver and stepping out of the car we contemplated our surroundings. What would lie behind the enclosure? Neil, our little guest, was allowed to buy the admission tickets and lead us to the entrance. As zoos go, it wasn't very big. Two sizeable rooms held about twenty large aquariums each with a snake and a sign.

We began with the first cage at the right of the entrance. A beautiful, patterned, green and red snake rested peacefully among the leaves. Edward realized that Neil couldn't read the information printed on the card so he did - out loud. "This beautiful snake lives on the floor of the forest and eats small animals that it catches. The bite of this snake can kill a small child." On to the next cage. Read the description which ended with: The bite of this snake can kill a small child.

Cage after cage. Same scenario. Look at the snake. Read its label. Always the same last sentence - The bite of this snake can kill a small child. Janet watched as Neil grew more and more agitated. She tried to signal Edward to not read those final words. He was oblivious. "Oh well" she thought. Only three more aquariums. We'll survive."

Two more done. There in the last cage, was a magnificent King Cobra. At the sight of the approaching people the serpent reared up high, hood flared, tongue darted in and out. All three, Edward, Janet, and Neil admired the glorious viper and Edward began to read. Habitat, life span, characteristics, routines all spewed forth and then the final sentence: The bite of this snake can kill a full grown man.

"Ooooooh" came from Neil, "but not a small child!"

Barry wanted to understand how it came to pass that she had diabetes and why this disease induced disintegration of vital body parts. Here she summarized information available through 1991.

Why?

Why does diabetes cause kidney failure? A good question. Unfortunately, there is no answer yet and when one is found, neither simplicity nor singularity will be characteristic. In other words there will not be one uncomplicated answer. Several explanations will interact. Currently, there are two main theories to explain why excess sugar in the blood causes damage. Both are probably involved. Maybe one process comes into play before the other. Maybe they happen at the same time. There are many things left to explain.

I'll pick one to talk about first. As a process, glycosylation is the attachment of glucose to a protein. Diabetics have heard this word because their glycosylated hemoglobin is measured to get an estimate of what their blood sugar control was in the previous two months. If there has been a lot of glucose in the blood, a lot of hemoglobin has been glycosylated and the value of the glycosylated hemoglobin is high. The new protein complex hangs around for a couple of months because red blood cells contain the glycosylated hemoglobin and two months is the life span of red blood cells. Another reason why glycosylated hemoglobin lasts so long is that its formation is an uncharacteristic chemical reaction. Most chemical reactions are totally reversible: A + B = AB happens just as fast as AB = A + B. By contrast the reaction: glucose + hemoglobin = glycohemoglobin is fast and glycohemoglobin = glucose + hemoglobin is slow. The quantity of glucose available is also quite important. If there is a lot of sugar, a large amount of glycohemoglobin in formed. Other proteins can be and are glycosylated in the blood stream and play a major role in causing diabetic complications.

Next question should be: How does glycosylated protein damage kidneys? Products of the next stage probably are responsible for sabotaging organs. Glycosylated protein molecules join together and form large clumps (aggregates). Sometimes these aggregates are so big that they can be seen under the microscope. (I know that you've been taught to think that things seen through a microscope are little but when molecules can be observed with the aid of this instrument they are *GIGANTIC* - for molecules.) Size alone can make physical problems. Thickening caused by their presence can make it difficult for substances to enter or leave structures. When big molecules stick to the walls of blood vessels, diameters are narrowed and blood pressure is increased. Moreover, this clumping process does not reverse so the aggregates of glycosylated protein remain and build up for a long period.

Now is the time to interrupt my tale of woe with a little hope. Recently, a drug (aminoguanidine) has been found to interfere with glycosylated protein aggregation and may even cause reversal. If these things are true, perhaps aminoguanidine can be used to avoid diabetic complications or even make them better once they have occurred.

If the second process explaining the bad effect of high blood sugar could be stopped it might eliminate the appearance of diabetic complications but probably could not reverse those that had already happened. Diabetologists know that glucose is converted within cells into another sugar, sorbitol, with the aid of the enzyme aldose reductase. Certain cells (kidney, retinal, and nerve) do not require the presence of insulin for glucose to cross their walls so when there is a large amount of sugar in the blood stream, there is much sugar inside these cells. The glucose converts to sorbitol which then is present in large concentrations. One of the major effects of sorbitol is that it causes microscopic edema (swelling) and problems due to cell enlargement. Myo-inositol is another chemical whose amount is dependent upon the quantity of sorbitol present. Exactly what myo-inositol does is unknown but it is believed to be tied up with energy production. Interference with the glucose to sorbitol pathway happens when aldose reductase inhibitors are given and there have been some successes with preventing diabetic complications.

Both of these processes, glycosylation and sorbitol production, result in raised blood pressure which is probably the major culprit in generating kidney disease in diabetics. So parts of an answer to the question "Why does diabetes cause kidney disease?" exist. Everything is not yet clear but we have strong hints. Maybe we shouldn't want to know the whole truth because if we did, think of all the researchers we would put out of work. Have pity on the rest of the world - not just the diseased parts!

In 1994, Barry took stock of her life as she did periodically. This time from the vantage point of someone who was present at the creation of kidney transplantation as a specialty both for training her spouse and for her own medical benefit. Here she tells of the medical giants she encountered along the way — specifically Adrian Kantrowitz— and how her hobby of document collecting was positively influenced by those she knew.

THANKS ADRIAN

Probably (no, not probably - absolutely), the best decision of my life was to say "Yes" to the young man. Four and a half years later we walked down the aisle but during that time he was accepted into medical school, attended, graduated, and was preparing to intern at the Peter Bent Brigham Hospital in Boston, Mass. Now, thirty-seven years later I look back in amazement at what I have lived through.

***

There are all sorts of ways to obtain an autograph. Mine can probably not be duplicated by many other collectors.

It was not purposeful, not calculated but made possible by my place in life (No - I'm not superior and don't claim to be.). I'm simply married to a well renowned physician who travels with the top people in his field. As a coat-tail participant I meet other well known physicians.

Thanks to my husband's success in his chosen field, I spent this morning sitting next to and talking with a Nobel Prize winner. (You can bet I have his autograph and because he is a gracious man, I possess photographs, personal notes, copies of some of his scientific papers, and his Nobel Prize address - all signed) Moreover, I had the pleasure of thanking him for my life.

No, I'm not being melodramatic. Dr. Joseph Murray performed the first kidney transplant between human identical twins and kept on working so that today, kidney transplantation is not considered an experimental procedure. My kidney transplant is almost fourteen years old. That makes me an unusual patient - I get to thank a man who has tangibally changed my existence.

But let's go on. Dr. Thomas Starzl, who is responsible for daring to use the combination of drugs which prevent my body from rejecting the foreign kidney is also a friend and yes, I have an ALS (Autograph Letter Signed) of his. One day he may be considered the surgeon of the century.

Willem Kolff, MD, inventor of the first practical artificial kidney is a dear, dear comrade. Last year we were in Kampen, Holland where he first used his device on the wife of an SS officer. He and I entered that historic room together and a photograph of our short amble, with an inscription to me, is among my prized possessions. Please note that I spent several months on dialysis. Thanks Pim, for my life.

The fourth man responsible for my breathing in and out every day is Belding Scribner, MD, another friend. In order to repeatedly use the artificial kidney, repeated blood stream access (about three times a week) is a necessity. If veins are punctured many times, they collapse and so useable sites wear out and no more dialysis can be done. Scrib solved that problem. His ALSs are marvelous. Important ones are hand written on yellow lined legal paper.

Not many patients share my joy in knowing these fellows but that is not the point of this story. I've rambled so you would understand the people I know.

Yes, I have their autographs but I've never seen one of them for sale in any catalogue. Maybe some day they will be, but meanwhile they remain my treasures.

In the meantime, total relaxation for me, is browsing through autograph lists, thinking about all the great people I can stand next to in my mind's eye. I daydream and then, one day, without warning, an autograph quote glared up at me. I know him! He knows me! Wait 'til I tell him. I waited.

This summer we were at a medical conference in Amsterdam, the Netherlands, honoring Willem J. Kolff, M.D. on the fiftieth anniversary of its initial use of the artificial kidney. During a reception in the Rembrandt Museum, I gazed around the room and saw him, Adrian Kantrowitz, standing in the middle of the room. Slowly, with inner glee, I approached. I had been biding my time, waiting to see him again.

"Hi Adrian. You're looking well. Do you know that your signature is for sale in autograph catalogues?"

"With a quizzical look, he laughed and said: "Oh, come on. Really?"

"Really. How much do you think you're worth?"

"Twelve dollars."

"Nope. Thirty five."

When I got home I realized that I had lied. Sanders *Price Guide to Autographs - second edition* claims a signature is $25, a signed document $68, and an ALS $145. Oh well, we all make mistakes.

We talked some more, looked at some masterpieces and parted company.

A few weeks later a letter arrived, addressed to me in script. Its return address was hand written as well. The note was personal. A gift to me from the surgeon who performed the first American heart transplant. Thanks Adrian.

Barry was a speaker at Willem J. Kolff's retirement/85th birthday celebration in Salt Lake City in 1995. These remarks are vintage Barry.

Ode to Willem J. Kolff

I have come to tell you a patient's story. It is the one I know best. It is mine.

We were married in 1957 and reported to the Peter Bent Brigham Hospital in Boston so Eli could start his internship. His first rotation was in the renal department. I was taken there to see the artificial kidney. In the room was a large, tub-shaped receptacle with a movable core that was carefully wrapped with sausage casing. Little did I think that that device would become an intimate part of my life. Diabetes reared its ugly head during a fourth pregnancy. We lost the baby but life went on. They told me the diabetes would disappear for many years but a few weeks after the delivery, I knew it was back. I was naive and uninformed about my disease. No worries about my medical future entered my mind. Ignorance, however, is not a protection.

The flu that was making me miserable wouldn't go away. At least, I thought it was the flu. Finally I was hospitalized and only hours later was presented with a choice: Get hooked up to the artificial kidney and begin dialysis or die. I had always protested the use of heroic measures to save lives but when the life was mine, I did a 180° turn and submitted to femoral needles.

This marvelous machine kept me alive for several months but because of my other diseases, dialysis was not the best treatment for me. A cooperative and loving, although not well matched, sister put me into the transplant program. The fistula in my arm was not used for very long but I wear it proudly.

Those months on the artificial kidney have given me 15 years, 15 exciting years. I have watched my 3 girls grow up, finish their educations (including graduate school), begin their careers, meet, fall in love with, and marry 3 (1 each) marvelous men, and fulfill a dream of mine. I never expected to hold a grandchild but now I have cuddled, rocked, fed, and changed 7.

I travel, I read, I write, I cook, I live.

Thank you Pim.

I have told you one story but there are thousands of stories out there. I'm going to tell you one more.

In our renal community there is a couple whom I admire. She was the girl Sam Kountz transplanted on nationwide television. The graft failed. Indeed, now she is on her third transplant. While enrolled in our dialysis unit she met a fellow patient, a man. It's unimportant but just so you can picture them - she is a small, always smiling, always chuckling black woman. He is a small, blind, diabetic Puerto Rican. They have been married almost 10 years and intermesh with each other in a wondrous manner. They obviously help each other but only when needed. He has had transplants too, but is currently back on dialysis. Now, this couple knows how important exercise is. They went to gyms, all of which rapidly turned them away: "Not here. Go away. Go away." We got them a treadmill. Recently they announced that they both have jobs. They work at their dialysis center (which for obvious reasons, is a good place for them to be employed). She is a clerk and he is being taught how to fix artificial kidneys.

Nothing keeps these people down but it is thanks to Pim Kolff that they go on.

A New What?" has a very happy ending is upbeat and educational throughout. As Barry reminisces: "There on the operating table, I expected an uneventful minor surgical procedure but a woman's world opened before me much like Edna St. Vincent Millay's universe expanded in front of her in "Renascence"." The National Writer's Club gave "A New What?" fifth place in their 1994 essay contest.

A New What?

I'm 57 years old and I have a new bellybutton. It's beautiful. Until I got it, I didn't know how much I missed the old one.

Missed the old one? How do you lose a bellybutton? Everyone has one. Well, about eight years ago, I developed an umbilical hernia which, by definition, was right in the middle of my belly. It wasn't big but that small outcropping of flesh did obliterate my bellybutton. This year it began to grow and I knew the time for fixing was at hand. Made arrangements and soon, there I was, stretched out on the operating table, arms extended, IV going, and my friendly surgeon, asking: "Do you want an inney or an outy?

Without a moments hesitation: "An inney. I just got rid of an outy."

And there it is - my brand new bellybutton. I contemplate it a lot. Many thoughts surround it, many feelings. The old one had been a flimsy physical connection with my mother, connecting us even through the space of death. All her love and care, her mistakes and accomplishments, her memory, her image, seemed packed into that small dent. When the old one left and then the new one appeared, my memories of her did not change, proving what I already knew: our continuing connection was in my mind and not in my bellybutton.

Strangely though, the other side, the inside side, sees joined to members of the next generation, to my children, my daughters. Oh I know that no real attachment exists between the bellybuttons of mothers and their children but I guess it's always been a fantasy of mine, an illogical belief. A sense of continuity, that we go on in an unbroken chain, bellybutton following bellybutton, dwells in my soul. Felt the same way when the fact of mitochondrial DNA burst into my awareness. Small bodies floating in the cytoplasm of each cell of higher life forms, mitochondria are important to the existence of the cell because they produce enzymes for important biochemical pathways. They're necessary to keep us alive. DNA is the stuff responsible for passing the codes of inheritance to descendants of whatever is reproducing. I was taught in college that DNA was in the nucleus of the cell. True, but there is more. For a long time it's been known that mitochondria also contain DNA. Today we look at that fact in a new light. Now we are beginning to understand that mitochondrial DNA may be very essential in continuing life.

Think. Human life begins when the sperm and egg unite but the sperm is basically a nucleus with a tail. Formed much like a whole cell, the egg contains maternal mitochondria. Fusing, the sperm and egg form a new life. At its very inception the new cell contains mitochondria. Mommy's mitochondria. We - women - have a greater percentage of input into each life than do men. Female mitochondria are passed along. What inheritance, what contributions to each new creature's physical form journeys on through maternal DNA, is not yet known. But when our daughters, have daughters a special bit of our inheritance (no matter how small) continues us. Sons dead end this uninterrupted DNA passage. Let's not put down boys. We need 'em. We love 'em but they can't pass on to their sons that little special piece of us.

I speculate on what it could be. Are maternal emotions based in physical features? Certainly motherly caring, the maternal instinct, and female drive to protect the young are alive in most women whether or not they have actually born children. Still, female DNA also passes to male children. Maybe activation depends on the environment (perhaps hormonal) peculiar to the "gentle sex".

I feel close to my girls. Closer still with this new knowledge. In a strange way I feel a bridge between me and *first woman* (Eve if you want or a Homo sapiens great, great, great, etc. grandmother).

Newspaper articles published recently speak of scientists feeling they could pinpoint *first woman* who lived way way back in the past. Somehow this intertwines with my reaction to Jurassic Park. No, dinosaurs don't have bellybuttons but they do have ongoing DNA. Cloning ancient creatures is only slightly possible but the DNA is still viable. If the DNA can be manipulated to form a whole animal, theoretically identical copies of the beast could be produced. Dinosaurs existed long before *first woman* but they reproduced sexually. They passed on maternal DNA. My feeling of history is long indeed.

Recent history is my daughters and their daughters. We share so much. We do so many things alike. We're women or will be women. And because of that, pregnancy probably will be or was, part of our lives. Pregnant, we're involved in the most intimate possible relationship. We're connected to a baby and that connection will physically end with the formation of a new bellybutton.

Maybe that's why I'm so happy to have one again. It's my joining with the past and with the future. My bellybutton.

Responding to her granddaughter who remarked about "Grandma's Wrinkled Behind," Barry wrote this self appraisal in 1994.

Ruthie

Yes Ruthie, my rear is wrinkled but I wouldn't have it any other way.

Yours is not. Yours is lovely and firm and pinchable and young. You like to watch me shower and I help you with your bath. Modesty doesn't exist between us. We think bodies are beautiful; that they speak of much.

My rear has crawled, walked, climbed, swum, roller skated, sledded, bowled, been loved, had babies and shared with me the many adventures of my life. Together we have walked along the Nile, seen the Taj Mahal, fallen off a camel, boated on the Seine, climbed the Great Wall of China, heard Aida at the baths of Caracalla, marvelled at Caesaria. We've looked at the single artifact left from the first Temple, Rembrandt, Picasso, Rodin's Thinker, the Pieta - there is only one for me - Mont Blanc from above, the magnificent waterfalls of the world, slums in South Africa. United we've climbed inside one of the pharaoh's pyramids, canoed on an African river...........and on and on.

We've raised three girls to be good people and beyond all our dreams, we've cuddled six grandchildren. Being alive to hold you, share thoughts with you, love you makes me appreciate the wrinkles and how I got them.

I wish you as wonderful a way of getting your wrinkles as I took and in the end a new little girl to marvel at them with love.

After considerable deliberation, this example of Barry's poetry is included as the closing remembrance of Barry. Nearly 20 years later, protecting her husband who collapsed from a gastrointestinal hemorrhage, Barry was able to be the "strong" marital partner just as she wished.

My Husband
9/17/77

Hear me! Oh my husband
How I adore thee
How I rejoice in thee
Giver of strength and love
Nourisher of me in myriad ways.

I cling to thee as I push away
Seeking footholds in the mire
I hurt thee as I stretch and
Reach to grow

My heart's desire
Is to be for thee
What thou art for me.

Hear me! Oh my husband
How I adore thee